CRUSADER WITH COMPASSION

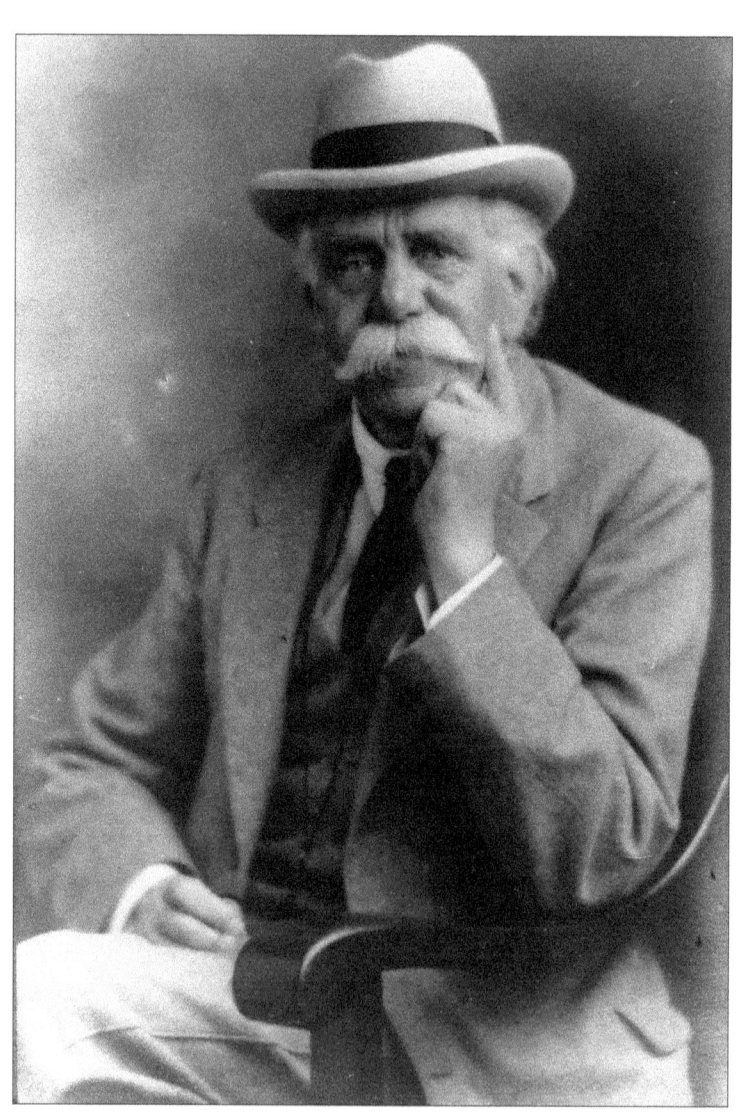

Crusader with Compassion

Dr Walter Hadwen
Gloucester GP
1854 – 1932

Dr Michael Till

First published in the United Kingdom in 2019

by The Hobnob Press,
8 Lock Warehouse, Severn Road, Gloucester GL1 2GA
www.hobnobpress.co.uk

© Michael Till, 2019

The Author hereby asserts his moral rights to be identified as the Author of the Work.

All rights reserved. No part of this publication may be reproduced, stored in a retrieval system, or transmitted in any form or by any means, electronic, mechanical, photocopying, recording or otherwise, without the prior permission of the publisher and copyright holder.

British Library Cataloguing in Publication Data
A catalogue record for this book is available from the British Library

ISBN 978-1-906978-78-5 (paperback)
      978-1-906978-79-2 (casebound)

Typeset in Scala 11/14 pt.
Typesetting and origination by John Chandler

CONTENTS

	Introduction	7
1	Hadwen's Origins and Development	9
2	Married Life	12
3	A New Era	27
4	Explanation of Conditions in Gloucester affecting the 1896 Smallpox Outbreak	43
5	Further challenges	56
6	Personal and Professional matters	68
7	Communication and Correspondence	73
8	John Hadwen, known as 'Jack'	83
9	The Great 'Smallpox' scare, 1923	92
10	Rex v Hadwen	103
11	Chillingham and Earl of Tankerville	123
12	The Traveller	128
13	Hadwen's Last Years and Death	133
14	Therapeutics	139
15	Succession	147
16	Postscript and Reflections	152

Appendices

1	Hadwen and Manslaughter Verdict, 1924.	158
2	Premature Burial	171
3	The Difficulties of Dr Deguerre	177
4	First Impressions of America	182
	Bibliography, Books and References	187
	Acknowledgements	190
	Index	191

Any royalty or copyright fees earned as a result of sales of this book will be donated to Rotary Foundation's Charity, 'End Polio Now'.

INTRODUCTION

Over the years I have collected many items about Dr Walter Hadwen. My collection of articles and documents has encouraged me to attempt a detailed record of his life. His years in Gloucester as a respected family doctor were preceded by taking a tortuous course from qualifying as a pharmacist and then on to gaining university entrance as a mature student to study medicine. He and his family had to make sacrifices to enable him to attend his studies at Bristol University and achieve this goal. This involved great personal determination, which is a hallmark of his character. His story shows just how his formative years really did influence his future career. He was a committed Christian and maintained his lifelong views as a teetotaller, vegetarian, and subsequently anti-vaccinationist and anti-vivisectionist.

Although the original biography *Hadwen of Gloucester* by Kidd and Richards is an excellent basic source of facts and quotes, its authors are hardly unbiased in their writings. The more I examined the profusion of publications and correspondence which Hadwen produced, the more difficult it became to give a clear and chronological outline of events. When I came to Gloucester in 1969 his name and fame were still a subject frequently discussed and remembered by his friends and patients with great fondness and admiration. Although his involvement in national causes increasingly occupied his time, his devotion to the care of his patients was his priority and the main reason for his decision to become a doctor.

This volume also includes a summary of one book for which he was responsible as editor. In addition, I have attempted to outline the content of two other books of which he was sole author. He achieved all this alongside campaigning articles in magazines and publicity pamphlets for all to read so that they could be appraised of the risk factors he believed would affect their health and lives.

His talent for preaching, both indoors and outdoors, and gift of oratory in public debate marked him as a lecturer and debater few could match. Inevitably his prominence as a speaker led to envy amongst his opponents and attempts were made to undermine his reputation. As time went on his dogmatic views led to much controversy. However, he defended his opinions by reading widely and analysing facts and figures to support his arguments and beliefs.

The demands on his time and energy to debate in public meetings must have impinged on his chosen professional life but the evidence suggests that he was willing to serve the needs of his patients at any time whatever the hour. At the most critical stage of his career, when he was challenged in court, not one patient left his practice and many members of the local population were prepared to show their loyal support and admiration for him publicly.

Gloucester was a busy city in which the docks were a centre of employment with associated engineering and a foundry. Importing of timber and grain transport on the canal system meant a demand for lower paid labourers. Dr Hadwen chose to practice, live and worship alongside these citizens and so had an understanding of their problems and aspirations. He fought for better living conditions and was successful in persuading the city authorities of their responsibilities in this respect.

Records confirm that his was a very full life, both here in his adopted home town, and time spent travelling to meetings elsewhere in England and further afield.

I hope my efforts will give more detail, information and insight into Dr Hadwen's life and the mark he left in Gloucester city. He has been described as one of the most influential personalities of his day, not only in this country, but in Europe and the USA.

Please read on and make up your own mind.

I
HADWEN'S ORIGINS AND DEVELOPMENT

IT IS POSSIBLE that the surname 'Hadwen' may be a derivation from a Danish name, but a detailed printed family history gives no hint of origin apart from the Carnforth area some eight miles north of Lancaster in the county of Lancashire. Hadwen's ancestors can be traced back to 1520 and the villages in which his forebears lived were noted to be all situated in that area.

Walter Hadwen's grandfather, Robert Hadwen (1791-1821) was a Lancastrian and solicitor. He married the 'belle of Lancaster', Dorothy Robinson, in 1816. In 1819 they had a son William Robinson Hadwen. By the age of two yrs, William was tragically orphaned, both parents dying in quick succession. Two uncles, who were partners together in a medical practice in Lancaster, took him under their care.

It is stated that his uncles arranged for him to be educated at Lancaster Royal Grammar School. More than one search in the school archives has failed to establish this fact and further enquiries by the local Family History Group do not confirm such a statement.

The plan was to encourage William to enter the medical profession but the sight of blood and screaming patients in his uncle's surgery revolted him and he ran away. Eventually he enlisted in the Royal Marines serving both at home and abroad for a few years. At the age of 30 years he settled in Woolwich where he was employed as a chemist and dispenser at the Royal Marine Infirmary. He married Sarah Pendle (1814-1910) from Suffolk and Walter Robert was their middle son, born 3 August 1854. The first son died aged seven years, the third son, John Henry, was born in 1857.

As Walter grew up, it is noted he was a prodigious scholar and could read Latin by the age of seven years. He benefitted from education by his father and the Infirmary chaplain. Having reached the educational standard required to gain entry to the Pharmaceutical Society he left school at the age of thirteen years. At this stage he became articled to a chemist in Powis Street, Woolwich where he had to support himself apart from his parents providing his clothing. He later wrote that he received no help, not even £10 from his parents, in the way of further assistance. He was an avid reader and read Dickens, Scott and Whittier as his favourites. He went to hear the evangelist Sir Arthur Blackwood preach in the open air. Blackwood was known to be a total abstainer and philanthropist.

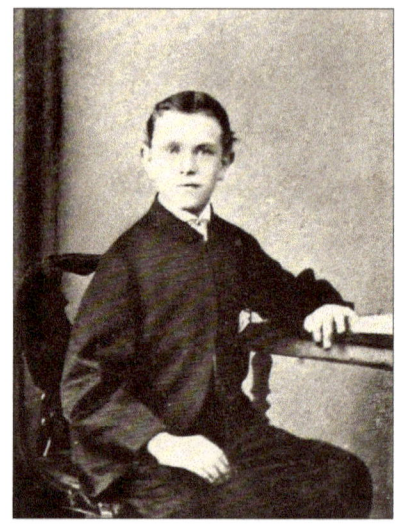

Hadwen aged 14 years

Walter's parents moved to Reading and left him in Woolwich in lodgings in 1869. The reason for this is explained by noting that the Royal Marines Woolwich Division disbanded after the closure of the Dockyard in 1869 and we presume William's employment ceased. He subsequently obtained a new position as dispenser at the Royal Berkshire Hospital in Reading.

As Walter matured he became interested in his appearance and attire. Photographs show that he always took care to present himself formally dressed. At this time he belonged to the YMCA and entered into discussion within the YMCA debating society whether females should be admitted to its membership. He is described as a 'man's man' and not a great admirer of the 'fair sex' as such. That attitude did change! There is also mention that he seriously considered following a friend to seek his fortune in Australia.

In 1872 , Walter moved to Bedford Square in London to work for another pharmacist. He had finished his contracted employment in Woolwich and the new post gave him more time to study and earn a small salary. Then, later, whilst employed as manager at a pharmacy in Clapham, it is noted that amongst the customers of the pharmacy were Charles Kingsley (1819-1875) and Mrs Catherine Dickens (1815-1879) wife of Charles and mother of his ten children.

Finally, later in 1879, he rejoined his parents in Reading where he worked for a John Wilson and was allowed more free time to complete his studies. It seemed his new employer was more than satisfied with Walter's assistance and indeed the business seems to have flourished. He passed his final examination for the Pharmaceutical College in April 1876 at the age of 22 yrs. The qualification was 'Licentiate Society of Apothecaries' L. S. A. This qualification allowed him to assist as pharmacist and dispense. At this stage of his life, Walter decided to follow his own convictions and firstly became a lifelong vegetarian, having witnessed the sufferings of animals taken for slaughter. He also joined the local Temperance Society founded by his father when living in Woolwich. His father is reported to have had an alcohol problem whilst serving in the Navy and resolved, for the sake of his family, to be a total abstainer. Hadwen also detested smoking.

He underwent confirmation whilst in Woolwich but his leanings were soon to be 'low church'! In 1875 he chose to join the Plymouth Brethren and started his evangelistic work, teaching and preaching, and eventually the gift of oratory served him well in many situations in his future life. While in Reading he decided to worship with the Plymouth Brethren and he saw first hand the schism developing within that organisation, but he persisted for the time being. However, he enjoyed the company of the congregation, mixing with old and young alike. He arranged days out by horse and carriage into the countryside with friends. The river provided exercise by means of of sculling. He was also a great walker, sometimes from London to Reading. Often, on walks, he was accompanied by his Welsh Collie called 'Fan'.

2
MARRIED LIFE

WALTER MET Alice Caroline Harral, who was the eldest child and daughter of Dr and Mrs Harral of Wimbledon. Alice was born in Jersey. Apparently this was love at first sight resulting in a whirlwind courtship of six months and they married in March 1878. Walter had great respect for Dr Harral, who practised homeopathy, and a close relationship followed. No description appears to be recorded of his wedding apart from the date, 26th March 1878 in Clapham. I have not discovered any photographs of the wedding.

In 1878 Walter and Alice decided to move to Highbridge, Somerset. No comment is made why this area was chosen and it may be that a suitable pharmacy business was advertised in a professional publication. Agreement to purchase was made.

According to the census it seems that the couple lived 'above the shop' and probably resided there as a matter of convenience in light of future developments. The address was 34 Market Place, Highbridge. The census at the time also shows that he had an apprentice pharmacist (Frederick Orchard) living in Hadwen's household in 1891.

He advised on human medical complaints and was known to perform dental extractions on his customers when necessary. On market days there was an influx of farmers and they sought Walter's assistance, not only for themselves but their animals as well. This activity matches well with his love and respect for all animals. The Somerset archives appear not to store images so there are no pictures available of the Market Place, (which later became Market Street), or of the pharmacy of that era. By the age of 24 years he had a flourishing business administering to the needs of human beings and the animal kingdom.

He planned and instigated the building of a Hall for Christian worship in Clyce Road and began open-air preaching, and soon was invited to other localities to preach. Such was his devotion that he even tramped one night a week to give lectures to a small community who met in a farmhouse.

His first baby, Una, was born in December 1879 and the law demanded the child be vaccinated (Vaccination Acts amended 1874). Walter investigated all the information recorded relating to side effects and other disease infection as a result of this preventative treatment. He resolved to resist this law at all costs. He appeared before the bench four times for baby Una, being fined a total of £50 with costs. This was followed in time by appearing in court three times for the same charge for his son, Jack, and then twice for his second daughter, Gracie. Apparently the bench gave up on continued prosecution. I have included a report from the *Weston Mercury* in 1882, Axbridge Petty Sessions. I have transcribed from a photocopy of the newspaper report and so there may be some minor inaccuracies. He was competent to defend his actions and this was not to be for the first time in his life.

There follows a copy of the proceedings of his prosecution. It demonstrates how adroitly Walter was able to defend his principles; and these long term principles were established and pronounced in public. The magistrates would have had to listen carefully to make a judgement.

Court case The Weston Mercury September 16th 1882
Axbridge Petty Sessions—extract

Rev. Yatman and Col. Colgrave, Magistrates.
Walter R Hadwen was summoned by the vaccination officer
Una Josephine Hadwen, under the age of fourteen years born 1879 has not been vaccinated and that you, the said Walter R Hadwen is the parent of the said child, and that the informant gave notice to you in writing requiring you, as parent, to have your child vaccinated within fourteen days thereafter and that the said notice has been disregarded.

Mr Hadwen is pleading not guilty and he has three reasons for so doing.

First, that the summons was illegal,

Secondly, that there was not a sufficient case against him upon the strength of the summons issued according to the 31st section of the vaccination Acts:-

The Magistrate's Clerk: Do you object to the process of the summons?

Mr Hadwen: I maintain it is an illegal summons.

The Magistrate's Clerk: You appear today and plead 'Not Guilty'?

Mr Hadwen: I am here to show cause why the complaint should not be preferred against me.

To the Magistrate's Clerk, Mr Hadwen admitted to the summons, that he was the father of the child mentioned in the summons, and that such child had not been successfully vaccinated. He then maintained that his reasons for disputing the legality of the summons were on the grounds that a similar notice had been served on him some time previously. He had been brought there and ordered to show cause to the Magistrates why he would not have his child vaccinated, and as he refused to comply with their order, he had to pay a penalty of 20 shillings and costs. He could however, show under the 31st section of the Vaccination Acts that he could not be brought up again before the Bench for a similar offence. Such a course was utterly illegal and it had been ruled as such by many authorities. There had been precedents in some courts where the second and third summons had been issued to parties for not having their children vaccinated, but such fact did not make the present prosecution legal. It was in his opinion, totally illegal and contrary to the spirit of the Act and the Law of Equity. Persons could not be summoned for the same offence twice, and he therefore maintained that the present prosecution was thoroughly illegal.

Lord Clifton had retired from the Bench because he was required to do so.

The Magistrate's Clerk: Lord Chief Justice Cockburn said it was perfectly legal.

Mr Hadwen: replied that in consequence of such opinion the current prosecutions were being instituted by the Boards of Guardians.

The Magistrate's Clerk then drew attention to the order of the Local Government Board as regards vaccination.

Mr Hadwen explained that Rev. Yatman had said on a previous occasion that the magistrates had nothing to do with the Local Government Board on the matter and that the justice acted independently of such authority. He added that the Lord Walsingham in moving the second reading of the Vaccination Acts 1871, amendment bill 1874, said it was in no way contemplated by this Bill to encourage prosecutions to the extent of persecution, but to leave a fair discretion to be exercised in case of conscious (conscientious)objection.

He (Hadwen) would therefore repeat that the present prosecution against himself was totally illegal, from the beginning to the end. He had paid the penalty for the offence in the first place and he considered it a disgraceful thing that a vaccination officer should summon him for an offence for which he had already paid the full penalty.

Rev Yatman: observed that as far as he could learn from the authorities, the Vaccination Acts implied continuous punishment

Mr Hadwen: if the vaccination acts are to be continuous punishment, then I must say, it is the most unjust and most iniquitous law ever passed. Precedence is no law, and a thousand wrongs will never make one right. According to the 31st Section, if a person does not have his child vaccinated and refuses to comply with the order of the vaccination officer, he is to be brought before the magistrates and if he disobeys this order he is to pay the penalty for the offence. Let the Bench show him any portion of the act which showed in any degree that they could bring him there for the same offence a second time.

Rev Yatman: I consider it legal.

Mr Hadwen then went on to say that ever since vaccination had been introduced into this country smallpox had increased. Smallpox, he explained, did not occur continuous, but it was an epidemic disease. There had been three great epidemics of smallpox since vaccination had been introduced which epidemics had been far greater than those previous to vaccination. In fact the last smallpox epidemic in 1881 was more terrible than had ever been known, being 122% higher than before vaccination was adopted. Let them take for instance, the case of Wednesbury in Staffordshire (now West Midlands). There, 79% of the children had been vaccinated and yet smallpox has raged to an awful extent in that place. Then again, fearful disclosures had been made in Norwich with regard to Smallpox. They also found from a deputation that waited upon Lord Cavendish, a short time since, that although the population had increased 10% smallpox had increased 120%. He would also draw the attention of the magistrate, not only in the increase in smallpox but more particularly to the more dreadful and fearful disease that was impregnated into children's blood by the poisonous lymph used. A return made by the medical department in 1877 showed that out of sixteen infants vaccinated at Misterton, Lincolnshire (now in Nottinghamshire), no less than six died within a month of erysipelas, which from a further return in 1880 was deduced the lamentable fact that, in round numbers, 4,500 infants under five years of age died in 1877 from syphilis, scrofula, skin diseases and erysipelas, more than the proportion of such deaths in 1877 would have given. If they examined the figures from the Registrar General in a return to the House of Commons in 1877 they would find that the deaths from syphilis amongst infants under 1yr had increased fourfold per million of births in 1875 compared with the returns of 1847. In 1847 the rate was 472 per million born, died of syphilis under one year. Whilst in 1875, 1, 826 per million born died of the disease under one year.

Rev Yatman: All these arguments have been brought before medical authorities and by large majorities they have decided vaccination is necessary, and therefore, what you have said is not a reasonable ground for abstention.

Mr Hadwen: There is another matter to which I would like to refer, and is one of the reasons why I do not have my child vaccinated. Does the compliance with the act of Parliament, as regards vaccination, prevent the spread of smallpox? I will have my child vaccinated if you can give me the stuff which will stop smallpox. I have written to the public vaccinator of the local government board and to five medical men, and I give it as evidence to this court that in each instance they have told me distinctly that they could not supply the stuff in accordance with the Vaccination Acts, viz. lymph that will prevent the smallpox. I now ask you to be supplied with pure lymph that does not contain the germs of disease. Erysipelas has increased fourfold, and syphilis has greatly increased, and as a parent loving my child, I dread the very thought of having such a child vaccinated with such conglomeration of filth as that obtained from the scabs and sores of beasts (Applause). Will the bench give me lymph which does not contain disease?

Rev Yatman: How many persons can have that?

Mr Hadwen: What right have you to enforce an Act of Parliament if you can't supply the stuff necessary for vaccination. The act of Parliament implies that a child is to be vaccinated so as to prevent smallpox and that consequently the lymph that produces the disease should not be used. It is one of the most distasteful and iniquitous Acts that has ever been passed. I feel exceedingly strongly upon the subject. It is a most cruel thing, and it is against the spirit of all true liberty. Under the circumstances, if you will order the Board of Guardians to supply me with the pure lymph, I will have my child vaccinated tomorrow.

Rev Yatman: We cannot do that.

Mr Hadwen: then how can you possibly order me to vaccinate my child when I cannot do so according to the Act of Parliament.

Rev Yatman: We make the order that your child shall be vaccinated within one month.

Mr Hadwen: You may fetch the money out of my pocket but my child shall never be vaccinated.

Parental summons to appear in court after refusing vaccination, within a notified time limit, in order to comply with the Vaccination Act 1867. This document is dated 1901.

In this report, Hadwen starts by saying he has three reasons for pleading 'not guilty', he mentions the first two points but legal arguments ensue and the 'third reason' is never specifically stated. No decision was recorded as to a punishment or fine in the newspaper report. However I have quoted the sum fined from his granddaughter's summary of the case.

Hadwen was a forceful orator, had knowledge of and could memorise statistics. Applause by his supporters is recorded twice in this report, so those present agreed with his views.

There followed further cases of parents refusing to have their child vaccinated, or not within the prescribed limit ordered previously by the Court or to pay the fine of fifteen shillings and sixpence. Different benches ordered fines of varying amounts, there was little consistency. The Anti-vaccination League was becoming very supportive to people who resisted vaccination and in some cases would pay the fines imposed. Hadwen had read papers by William Young, who at that time, was secretary of the League and their 'mouthpiece' was the *Vaccination Enquirer*. Originally the League was formed in 1866 and underwent various changes and addresses becoming a national force. It was renamed the National Anti-Vaccination League in February 1896 with the following objectives:

> To repeal the Vaccination Acts; the disestablishment and disendowment of the practice of vaccination; and the abolition of all regulations in regard to vaccination as conditions of employment in State Departments, or admission to Educational, or other institutions - later adding the vindication of the legitimate freedom of the subject in matters of medical treatment.

The *Vaccination Enquirer* publication was established by William Tebb FRGS in 1879, and his name will be mentioned later in Hadwen's story. Although there are many pamphlets associated with this movement I have not found proof that Hadwen contributed directly to their content and no indication that he was appointed to hold office within the organisation.

Generally anti-vaccinators were fined heavily and if unable to pay were imprisoned. There were groups in Weston-Super-Mare who clung to their convictions and were sent to jail in Bristol. By 1898 the Act was further amended and penalties removed. (The city of Leicester was also a renowned hot bed of anti-vaccinators.) Hadwen was very open and public about his views in this respect.

A son, John (known as Jack) was born in 1883, Gracie was born in 1886. Another child, William was born in December 1881 and died two months later of bronchopneumonia. None of the children were vaccinated.

An unrelated episode brought him before the bench, also in 1882, when he was sued by a customer whose dog got behind the pharmacy counter and ingested some poison and died. How Hadwen defended himself is recorded in an extract from the *Weston Mercury and Somersetshire Herald*. Again, it illustrates how Hadwen could conduct and defend himself in court.

Report on Appearance in Court on Dog Poisoning Case.
Weston Mercury and Somersetshire Herald June 30th 1882

The case was brought when an itinerant Theatrical Proprietor claimed £6 from the defendant, a chemist, Mr Hadwen of Highbridge, for the loss of his dog from taking poison on the defendant's premises, Mr Brice, who represented the plaintiff, said his client had recently opened a temporary theatre in the vicinity of the defendant's shop. He had gone into the shop to purchase mixtures. The dog followed him into the shop and got into a place behind the counter. Unfortunately Mr Hadwen or his assistant had placed poisoned bread with a view to killing vermin. No precautions had been made. The valuable dog was lost (died). The dog was a retriever. He accused the owner of carelessness. It was said that more dogs may have been so affected. Unsubstantiated evidence was given on this point. The dog was not chained and did not require it! Mr Hadwen gave specific detail as to when and wherein the shop the bread was placed. The piece of bread would have only been reached by a dog on its hind legs. The rear of the counter was not for public access. The assistant, when he realised what had happened immediately removed the bread from the dog's mouth and the bread removed from the shop and the dog did not appear to be any worse for the occurrence. The bread had only just been taken out of a drawer and put out of the way to be destroyed and to be replaced with fresh bread with poison as mice did not like stale bread. The dogs which came into the shop had been a great nuisance and had spoiled a lot of his goods.

The judge stated that if a person took his dog into chemist's shop, where there are all sorts of things necessarily exposed, he did so at his own risk. The dog had not been invited into the shop. The defendant was not responsible in this instant.

Judgement in favour of the defendant was awarded with costs.

It is obvious that Hadwen's activities never stopped and in 1884 he experienced a 'breakdown of health' and took a holiday with his wife to Antwerp, Brussels, Luxembourg, Basle and Berne. Hospitality was offered by local Plymouth Brethren.

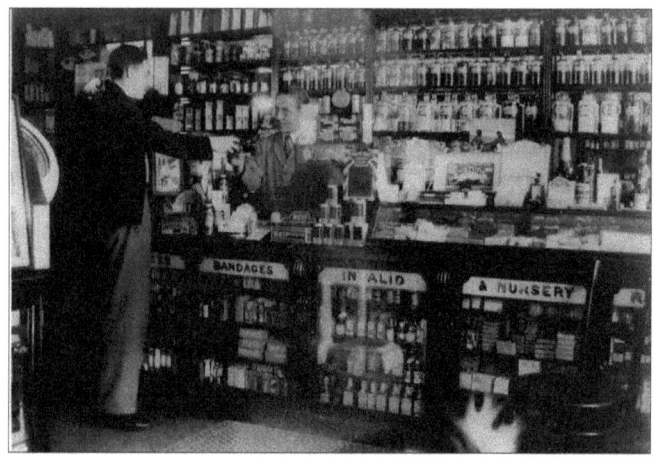

Typical Pharmacy in Highbridge early 1900s (not 22, Market Street)

It would seem that Hadwen's Pharmacy was a very successful business and he was widely respected for his advice to parishioners. However some dissatisfaction about his future personal professional role began to emerge and he planned to apply to Bristol University to obtain a degree in Medicine.

It is stated, in one report, that once qualified and practising as a family doctor back in Highbridge, he disposed of his Pharmacy. His premises were at 22, Market Street. I have checked this out with local historians and pharmacists as there were other similar businesses in the same street. A retired pharmacist informed me he worked for a Fred Orchard, Chemist at 36, Market Street and this can only relate to the same named person living with Hadwen when an apprentice. A later owner of the 22, Market Street premises was a Bell Kidd, then John Chanon, MPS. who sold on his 'Hills Pharmacy chain' to Lloyds

Pharmacy Group. This is as accurate a history of the outcome of the premises at 22, Market Street as I can ascertain.

Besides the academic challenges there must have been many other sacrifices for him and his family. One assumes that he had a trusted apprentice pharmacist who could look after the business in his absence. He probably had some financial support from his father-in-law and his parents moved from Reading to 4, Sunnyside, Burnham so that his father could also oversee the pharmacy business. He had his wife's support although she had the responsibility of the family and according to the census return there were two servant girls in residence in the home.

His first disappointment was that his qualification in Chemistry was insufficient to satisfy the requirements for entry into the medical faculty and he had to resit an exam in this subject. He also had to prove his knowledge of Algebra, Geometry and Mechanics to obtain the Medical Student's Registration Certificate at the office of the Medical Council, London which enabled him to join the Bristol University Autumn Session in 1888.

He had to travel to Bristol by train and this proved impossible to get to lectures in time for 9am. The only solution was to travel to Bristol on the last train at night and sleep over in rooms rented in Bristol. He arrived back at his home by 5 o'clock and attended to business and correspondence as well as two Bible Study evenings per week in the Clyce Road Hall and then completed his medical studies. It was back to Bristol last thing at night. After three years he took up temporary residence in London for the purpose of taking his degrees in Surgery at St Bartholomew's and studying midwifery at Queen Charlotte's Hospital. He had a short holiday with his wife in Paris in 1891 but apart from that he had no break from studying or his commitments in Highbridge. He qualified M. R. C. S. (Eng.), L. R. C. P. (Lond.).

His achievements, as a student, were to be awarded as reported from the University archives:-

1888	Winter Session, Junior Class of Anatomy, Certificate.	
	Junior Class of Physiology, Certificate	
1889	Winter Session, Senior Class Anatomy, Certificate	
	Senior Class Physiology, Certificate	
1890	Winter Session, Medicine, Certificate	
	Surgery, Certificate	

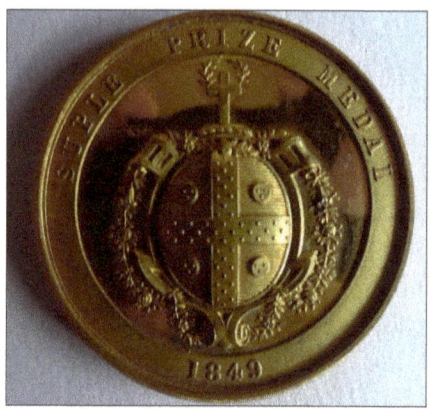 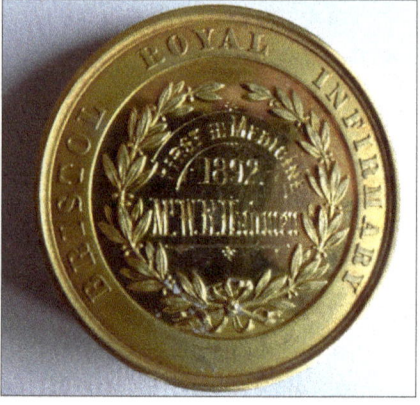

The Suple Prize Medal, 'First in Medicine' Mr W.R.Hadwen, 1892

              Clark Prize for Student in 3rd year who has most distinguished himself in Class Examinations. Prize value, 15 guineas
              Suple Medical Prize, a gold medal & Prize value 7 guineas
1891-92 Summer Session Operative Surgery, Prize
              Pathology and Morbid Anatomy-Certificate
1892-93 Winter Session Pathological Prize for proficiency in Pathology & Morbid Anatomy Prize value 3 guineas.

His final qualification was to obtain an MD Degree at St Andrew's confirmed by the following letter:

Thank you for your enquiry about Walter R Hadwen and his award of MD in 1893. We have a publication, the *Biographical Register of the University of St Andrews 1747-1897* and his entry reads:-

Hadwen, Walter Robert MD 26-Mar-1897 by examination. Born 3-Aug-1854 Studied Bristol and St Bartholomew's hospital MRCS Eng. 1893 when he was from Highbridge, Somerset LRCPL 1893. LSA 1893. Practised Gloucester. Anti-vivisectionist. President, British Union for the Abolition of Vivisection. Publications. Died 1932

One of the sources quoted for this entry is a book by B E Kidd entitled *Hadwen of Gloucester, Man, Medico, Martyr* which was published in 1933. You probably already know this book. But you will see that there is a discrepancy with the dates. Our records show that the award of MD was made in 1897.

The following is extracted from the Minutes of Senatus for 1897:

25th March 1897: An adjourned meeting of the Senatus Academicus was held this morning at 9. 40 o'clock for the purpose of opening the

Medical Examinations.

It was reported that 13 candidates being Registered Medical Practitioners above the age of forty years whose professional position and experience had in each case been vouched for by not fewer than three Medical men of acknowledged repute in their profession had presented themselves for examination for the Degree of M. D.

It was agreed that the examinations should begin at 10 o'clock and continue till 1 o'clock; and resume at 2 o'clock and continue till 5 o'clock; also that they should be resumed tomorrow morning at 8 o'clock and continue till 11 o'clock.

The adjourned meeting resumed the next day, the 26th of March, and received reports from the various faculties on the examination results prior to holding Graduation. The report of the Faculty of Medicine reads:

Professor Pettigrew reported on behalf of the Faculty of Medicine that the following Registered Medical Practitioners of above the age of forty years had following Registered Medical Practitioners of above the age of forty years had passed satisfactory examinations in the following departments of Medicine

1) Practise of Medicine 2) Surgery 3) Midwifery and the Diseases of Women and Children 4) Materia Medica and Medical Jurisprudence, and we recommend for the Degree of MD:-

There follows a list of 10 names, the fifth being Walter Robert Hadwen, Gloucester.

His entry in the list of candidates for the MD gives his address when he applied in 1894 as, 34 Brunswick Square, Gloucester. He was recommended for the degree by: W H [Narsant or Narsaut] FRCS, Bristol; R S Smith MD, Bristol; WS Collins M. S. MD, BSc, London. I have bracketted 'Narsant/Narsaut' as this is my best guess at the name. The hand is not the most legible. Similarly it does appear to be M. S. that follows Collins' name.

In the 18th and early 19th centuries the MD could be awarded 'by testimonial' when the candidate only had to submit recommendations by medical men

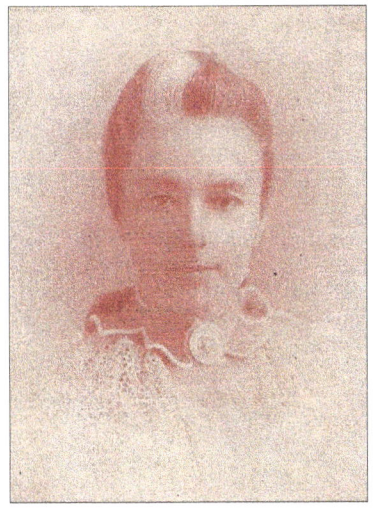

Mrs Hadwen-Undated

of good standing, recognised by the University. The testimonials would bear that the applicant was of good standing and character, had sufficient experience and had attended courses of instruction at recognised institutions or under eminent men. If Senatus were minded to accept these testimonials, the degree was awarded, often without the candidate coming anywhere near St Andrews. By the mid-nineteenth century this was replaced by the examination which gradually became more exacting, taking place over several days. In 1897 new regulations were put into place that brought the study of medicine more into line with other science degrees.

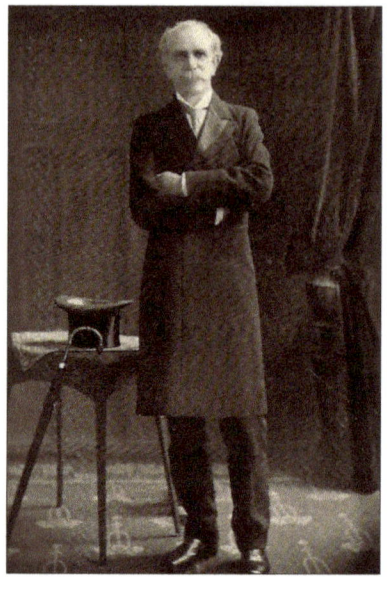

Dr. W. Hadwen - Undated

John S G Blair, *History of medicine in the University of St Andrews* (Edinburgh, Scottish Academic Press, 1987) gives an excellent overview of the faculty and the ways in which degrees were awarded. He also explains the the political climate that made a Scottish degree the only option for many English practitioners. Interestingly, on p. 155 he notes that the second most important medical event in St Andrews University of 1897 was the last examination for the MD under the old regulations. This occurs on 26th March as above and he lists the graduates. Walter Hadwen is, therefore, mentioned in this work. The most important thing that year, according to Blair, was the new Bute Medical Building which was still in use until about a month ago when the new medical building (as yet un-named) was opened. The Bute building was named after the Lord Rector of the University at the time, the 3rd Marquis of Bute, who endowed it.

From the information we have, Hadwen qualified as a doctor in 1893 and returned to Highbridge to practice as a family practitioner. As the letter from St Andrew's states there is this discrepancy in dates as to his MD which seemingly will remain unresolved but does not alter the fact that the qualification is confirmed after he moved to Gloucester rather than while resident in Highbridge. Later in his medical career there was an accusation that there was doubt over his qualification as a doctor and that is why there is detail here confirming his attendance and qualification at medical school. Many doctors, writing in Hadwen's time, seemed to show their medical qualification including M. D.

Having expended much energy, both mental and physical, in completing his medical qualification, a holiday was arranged in 1884, before his second daughter (Grace) was born. He travelled with his wife from Harwich to Antwerp and attended a Health Exhibition. From there they ventured to Brussels, Luxembourg, Basle, Berne, Lucerne. He undertook long 12 mile walks on some days.

Altogether Hadwen was in Highbridge for over eighteen years and is credited with campaigning to improve the sanitary conditions (sewerage and fresh drinking water) for the townsfolk resulting in a healthier lifestyle. He also campaigned to improve road conditions to make travel safer.

Although many areas in UK were constantly affected by outbreaks of smallpox, there is no specific mention of severe outbreak in Highbridge. However, his views as an anti-vaccinationist were becoming widespread throughout the South West and a group in Gloucester with similar views approached him for assistance. He addressed public meetings there which were attended by large numbers who held anti-Jennerism views. This group argued that the city authorities had neglected the state of sewers and sanitation and this was the cause of the smallpox outbreak. Hadwen came in support, visiting the city several times to obtain a factual insight into the health problems in the city. He apparently visited and inspected the 'local hospital' and also patients' homes.

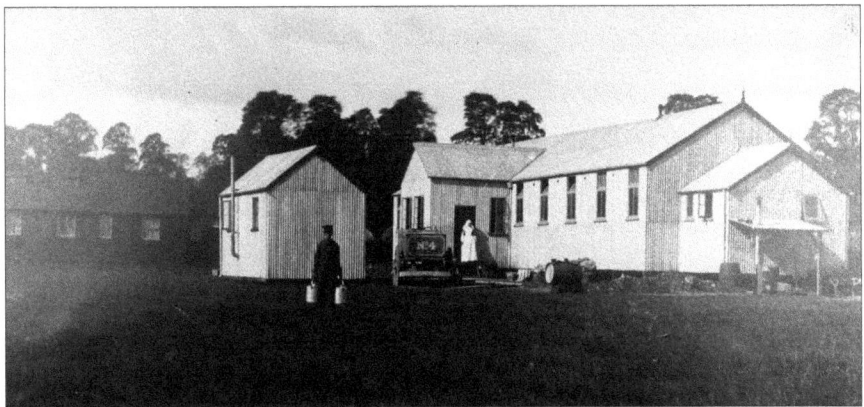

Wooden buildings of Isolation Hospital on the Lannet, possibly showing a milk delivery, water bowser and uniformed nurse (undated).

The hospital he almost certainly visited was the Isolation Hospital sited on the Lannett off King Edwards Avenue in Gloucester, now a recreation and rugby field. The hospital unit was purchased in 1874 from the Cheltenham Improvement Commissioners. Originally of wooden construction providing only fourteen beds, it was later enlarged and by 1888 was largely constructed of brick. A detailed report in 1897 describes the deplorable conditions in this amenity when inspected. This facility was closed in 1903 and transferred to Field Farm, near Longford. The new Over Hospital was not opened until 1903 and was to treat all infectious diseases not just smallpox.

After the smallpox epidemic waned, a manifesto was sent to Hadwen signed by over a thousand citizens, begging him to leave Highbridge and establish himself in practice in Gloucester.

As he left Highbridge there were meetings of friends and colleagues who expressed their thanks for his services to the community and various presents were offered.

He made the move to Gloucester, with his family, in October 1896.

3
A NEW ERA

IN BEGINNING this new phase in Hadwen's life, we have to try and fill in a little of the background to the medical and political situation that pertained in Gloucester in 1896. The authorities had declared the smallpox epidemic over by June of that year but the aftermath was a time of blame and debate on how the health of the population was to be protected in future.

Despite being a mature qualifier in medicine, including a pathology prize, Hadwen was consistent in his view that vaccination and vivisection were abhorrent. His strong personality expressed his views both in public and also many articles and publications, that vaccination was not the answer to the epidemic. Health was improved by better housing, and improved sanitation and drinking water were his mission. This convinced the populace that the city had failed its inhabitants by allowing the disintegration of the sewerage and drainage facilities and an inadequate supply of good quality drinking water. Again, his strength in argument was in using statistical evidence to support his theories.

The generally accepted 'germ theory' and the evidence that white blood cells could kill germs was not one with which Hadwen agreed. This was Metchikoff's theory publicised in the late 19th century. Indeed he held in contempt such a proposition. An understanding of bacteria and viruses was not universally accepted when he started his work as a GP. Antibodies and their part in disease resistance was yet to be recognised. Jenner's invention and Jennerism were an anathema. In reading about progress in medical science at this stage it appears that Europe was ahead in accepting the germ theory and UK and USA were slower to affirm it.

The politics locally involved the city councillors and also the Poor Law guardians who generally proved to be against vaccination and in particular the 1873 Act. There was concern that vaccination was a risk from impurities and may be a source of transmitting other diseases like syphilis. Compulsory vaccination was also considered an infringement of civil liberty. Statistics were unreliable but one shows that in the city there were 2, 035 cases of smallpox in 1896 with 446 deaths and much residual morbidity. It was claimed that of those deaths 25% had been vaccinated.

The council had failed to appreciate that the provision of isolation hospital facilities was totally inadequate, originally with only fourteen beds. A very small 'Cholera Hospital' existed and is mentioned later. In 1896 it is recorded that there were 150-300 new cases of smallpox per week, so facilities were totally inadequate. Many cases were therefore treated at home and this resulted in infected children sharing beds, thus spreading the contagious disease further. A Royal Commission investigated the anti-vaccination grievances but took seven years to publish its findings in 1896. Hadwen's views also affected the argument in that he was against the introduction of material sourced from animals and any animal experimentation.

In 1897 a Local Government Board grant of £4,000 was received to improve drinking water and sewerage facilities, all too late. The building of Over Isolation hospital, just outside the city, only started in 1897. Statements were made that 'the contagion of smallpox was spread through effluvia from the drains' in line with the miasma theory. The local medical officer of health at the time however stated 'cess pools and foul drains convey germs and lower residents' vitality'

Hadwen is said to have suggested that the anti-vaccinationists burn an effigy of Jenner at the next Guy

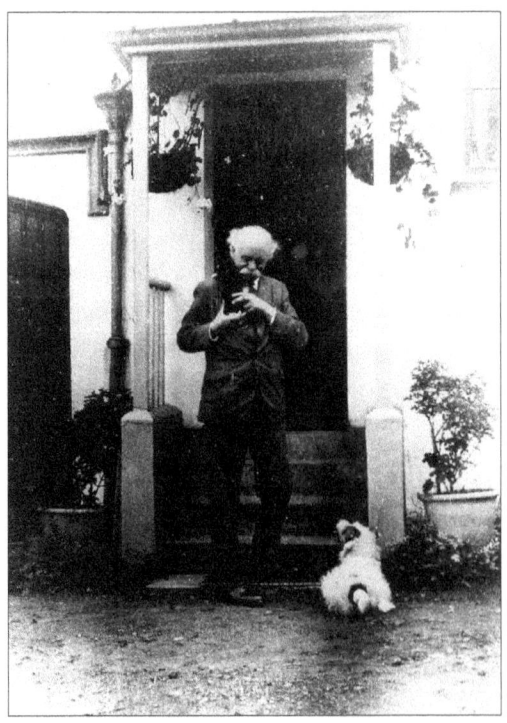

Hadwen outside 'Brunswick House', Brunswick Square, Gloucester

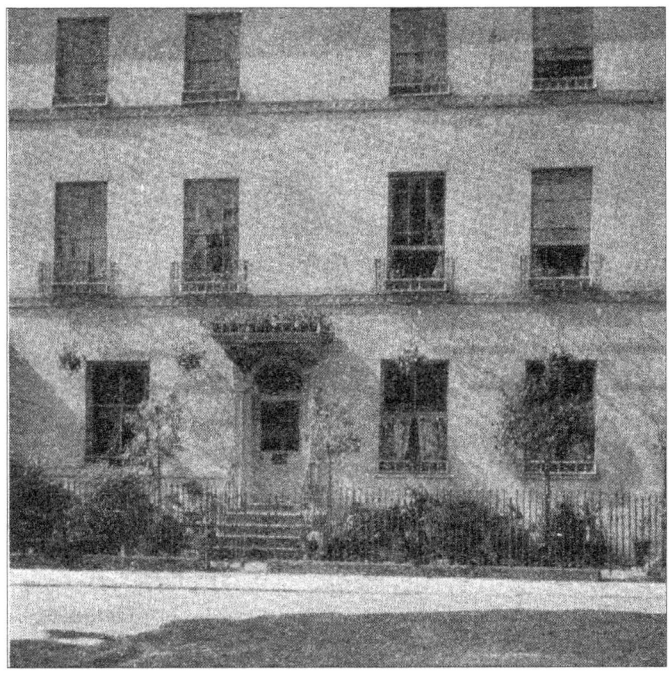

Brunswick House at time of Trial, the plate on the door of house bore the inscription W.R. Hadwen. M.D.

Fawkes celebration! However, Jenner is now honoured by a statue in Gloucester Cathedral in recognition of his contribution to world health.

So this is the background to the atmosphere in Gloucester as Hadwen settled into a new home and practice.

As always, one would like to be able to clarify detail on many points about a historic figure, but inevitably there is uncertainty. Hadwen bought his house and moved into it in October 1896. The house was named in correspondence as 'Brunswick House' in Brunswick Square in the city Centre. On redevelopment of the south side of the square the numbering was revised. One original document gives the number as 35. As far as we know this was a family home and not used as a regular surgery for consultations. His children appeared to be happy and they had a house keeper, Mary, who looked after them kindly and of whom they were very fond.

Patients would know the address and call directly for help as there is no evidence of Hadwen having a telephone in his early years in Gloucester. We also have to assume that he rented, rather than owned, his surgery premises at 139, Barton Street. By 1918 personal notepaper shows a telephone number '106' !

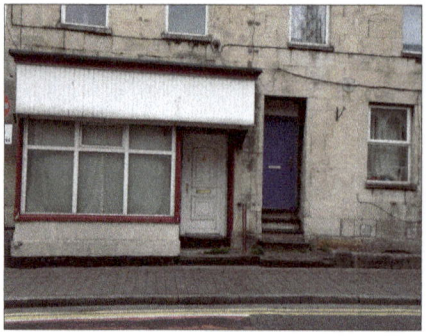 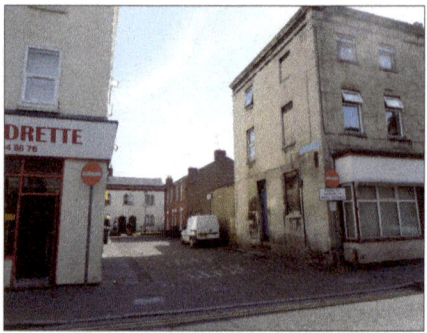

This photo of the present state of the entrance door (blue) to the surgery also shows the adjoining shop premises owned by Duckworths in 1970 and now in disrepair

Nicknamed 'The Umbilicus' with the old Duckworth Pharmacy on right in Barton Street and the cul-de-sac approach to Gothic Cottages at the rear.

There are reports of Hadwen founding Hydropathy Society facilities in Highbridge, and on arrival in Gloucester he was quick to join in the inauguration of the Gloucester Medical and Hydropathic Association. A few years later he was able to purchase the adjoining property to his house in Brunswick Square to make a single property and create a centre for hydropathic and electric treatment. His daughter, Grace, trained and practised as a masseuse and used these premises. Strict vegetarian advice was given. Grace carried on until she married in 1913. After that date the house reverted to being a family private residence.

The following information was given to employees of the local company

Matthews and Co. Ltd. , High Orchard Works

Gloucester Medical and Hydropathic Association has been established to provide Medical and Surgical attendance for those who are pecuniary unable to obtain it in the ordinary way and advance the principles of Hygiene and Hydrotherapy. Members consist of Honorary Subscribers of ten shillings and six pence and upwards annually and Benefit Members above fifteen years, who pay one shilling per quarter and children of the Benefit members who pay six pence per quarter. Benefit members must be in good health on joining, and are admitted free to all lectures. '

Secretary-Mr W. Heard of 11, Herbert Street, Derby Road.
Medical Officer- Dr Walter Hadwen, 35, Brunswick Square
Surgery-139 Barton Street. Hours 9-10am and 6-7 pm

At this time also local opinion prevented the use of the East End Tabernacle in Derby Road, Gloucester as a hydropathic hospital. The application for such use was by J. N. O. Pickering who worked in Gloucester with his 'Water Cure' for which he made great claims (see bibliography). His booklet mentions having patients attend him in Clement Street, Gloucester, but no detail of how the water cure was administered or performed. The only minor information mentioned was that the water was treated with Permanganate of Potash.

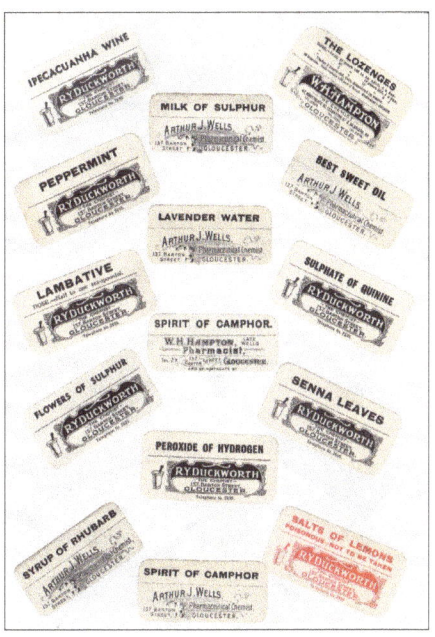

Duckworth's, Wells and Hampton's Pharmacy medicine labels. (typical early 20th century)

I arrived in the Practice in October 1969 when Barton Street surgery was still used as a branch surgery near to what had been developed as a main surgery at 25a Park Road, Gloucester. The photograph shows an entrance door with at least four steps from the footpath, with no rail or bar to assist the infirm patient. The door led directly into the small waiting room. I doubt that Hadwen had a receptionist. A door led through to a consulting room with just enough space for a desk, a couple of chairs and couch, a basin with running cold water (an electric hot water heater was installed after Hadwen's time). There was a connecting door to the Pharmacy shop next door (Duckworth's, 137, Barton Street). I assume Hadwen, with his pharmacy qualification, was able to prescribe and dispense commonly used medication from bulk containers, but no doubt used the adjoining chemist for further supplies.

There was another doctor's surgery at 141 Barton Street, a Dr Graham and I believe his son followed in his father's practice there in the 1970s. Around the corner from the surgery was 'Gothic Cottages' whether still used for isolation of Cholera at that time or other infectious diseases again is never mentioned in Hadwen's documents. Apparently, in its day fouled linen was kept in non-functioning baths, and excreta burned on ground very near the building. The water was supplied via

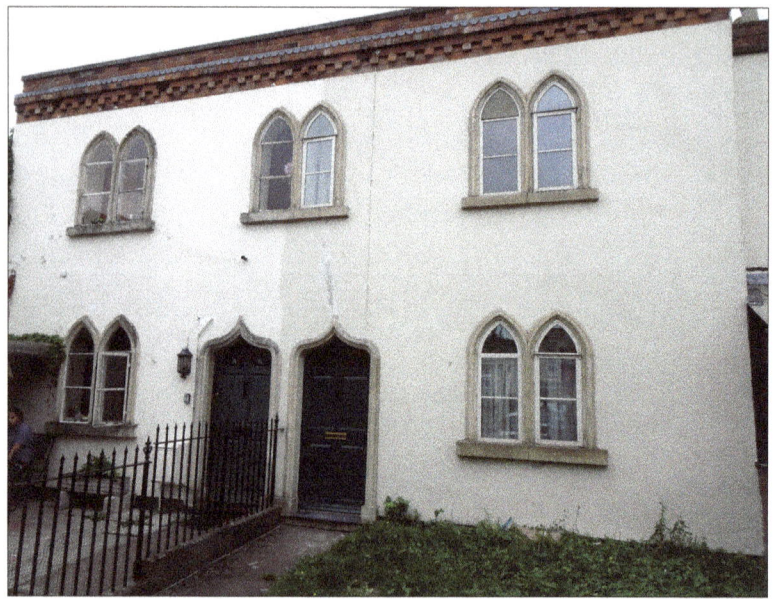

Gothic Cottages as they stand today, the right hand cottage has been restored to a high standard.

horse and cart with a water bowser. There was no drainage. The present owner of the property told me he was led to believe that where there is now a brick wall, on the left, as you approach the cottages, this was the site of a small mortuary.

There exist various descriptions of Hadwen's appearance and character. He had twinkling blue eyes, his original good crop of tawny hair was beginning to grey until, in later life, it became snow white. All images show his formidable moustache. He was a man of indomitable spirit with a deep faith, buoyant and optimistic and said to be tolerant but did not suffer fools lightly. When tired and stressed he displayed a harsh temper. His voice was described as warm and vibrating. He was an inveterate correspondent and there are examples of his sketching talents.

The story goes that Hadwen (top bunk) was with Alderman Fielding (bottom bunk) on a 'voyage' and in the middle of the night Fielding thought he heard the scratching of mice in the sleeping area only to discover that Hadwen was deep in correspondence and it was the scratching of a pen he had heard. Alderman James Fielding was the MD of Fielding & Platt who had their major Atlas works on the quayside from 1866 to 1966. He would have been a compatible companion for Hadwen as he was a Liberal, Puritan and nonconformist.

When Hadwen commenced working in practice he could only afford a push bike, but then progressed to a motor bike and eventually a smart motorcar. Thursday was Gloucester's half day closing, and still was into the 1960s. He used this spare time to explore on foot or bike the surrounding area with his children.

He claimed he was never wealthy but was generous with his own money but prudent with monies donated to official causes. Apparently he never agreed to a fee for any of his public lectures and insisted on travelling only third class. He once applied for the post of medical officer for the city and was acknowledged as the best qualified applicant, but the decision was made in favour of another applicant as it was stated Hadwen spent too much time out of the city. £100 annual income was lost. He was an accomplished orator and public speaker. All his best talents would come into play at various stages of his future life.

The local medical profession were outraged by his views and no doubt by his popularity; for them he was a social outlaw. A meeting of local medical men, encouraged or even coerced by British Medical Association members, is said to have pledged to 'run him out of town' within six months, and he was never welcomed at any BMA meeting. However, this does not seem to have deterred him from much correspondence with the *British Medical Journal* which will be mentioned later.

As regards his religious faith, he had shown an empathy with the Plymouth Brethren but once established in Gloucester he decided that a more independent gathering of worshippers was more to his taste.

Copy of marriage certificate dated 1929 and signed by Hadwen, ceremony taking place at Albion Hall

He had already preached in St. Mary's Hall in 1897 (it had been an old theatre but now demolished), then he re-located to the 'Old Institute' and moved again renting rooms in Glevum Hall, a small concert hall above premises, all in Southgate St. A member of this congregation owned three cottages in Southgate Street and offered them for the construction of a larger meeting house. An architect friend of Hadwen's designed the building with amenities near the entrance and the worship area built at the rear on the gardens of the cottages. Albion Hall came into being in 1906 and is now known as the very active 'Southgate Evangelical Church'. In 1921 Hadwen handed over the ownership of the Hall to trustees.

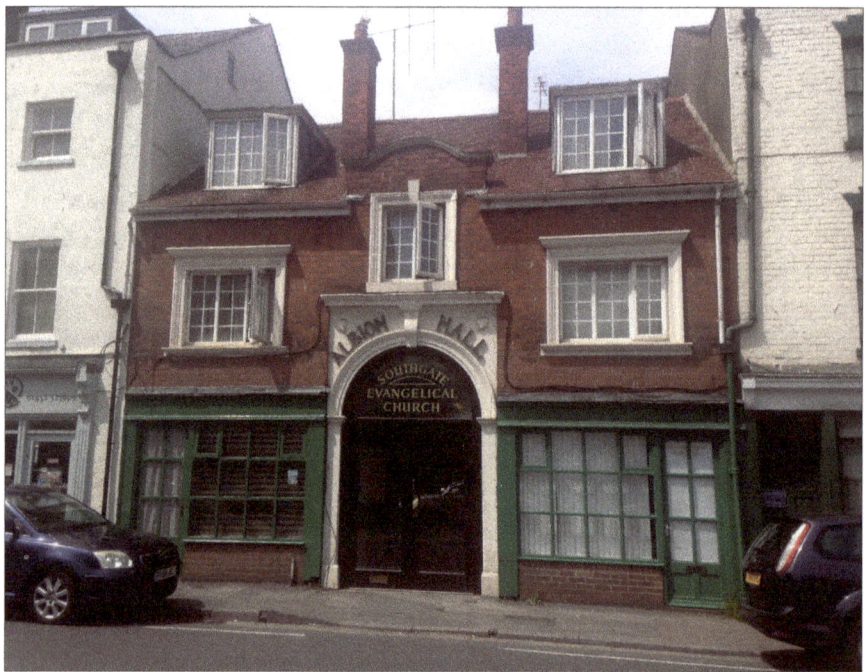

Albion Hall, as it stands today in Southgate Street, Gloucester, now preferring to use the title 'Southgate Evangelical Church' with a very active congregation

Three hundred children attended Sunday School encouraged by prizes for attendance and an Annual Summer outing. A Band of Hope was started to encourage abstinence. Hadwen ran preparation classes for those intending to become full members of the Assembly and he preached most Sunday evenings, advertising the subject of his sermons in the local press. The breaking of bread was celebrated with Hadwen officiating. The Hall became licensed for the solemnisation of marriages in 1913. Hadwen was the Officiating Minister or Registrar and he himself married his daughter, Grace, to Eric Newman. In 1916 he printed a 58-page booklet *The institution of the Lord's Supper. Its Observance among early Christians.*

Eulalie, Hadwen's granddaughter, recorded that as a girl she was instructed to attend the evening service at Albion Hall when her grandfather was preaching or forsake her supper!

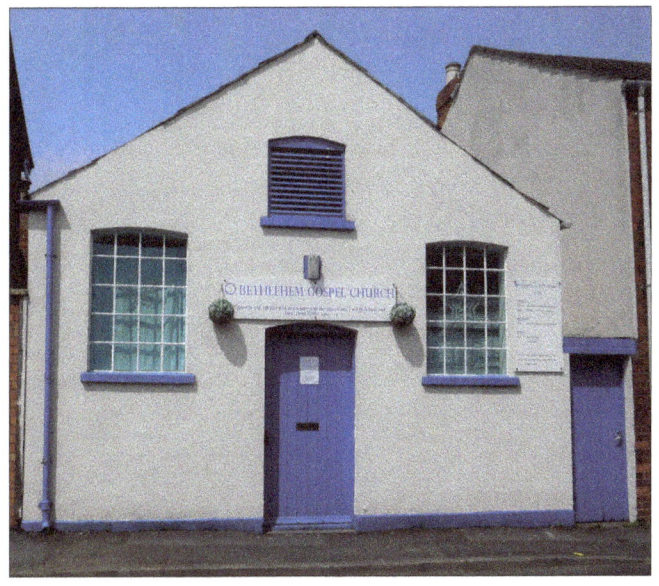

The Mission Hall, Nelson Street, Gloucester

The mission hall in Nelson Street, bought by Hadwen from a building company, was owned by him until his death when, in his will, he transferred ownership to the Albion Hall trustees to assist its future witness in the area. This is still the case, and the hall has a congregation of around 35 worshipers and a pastor in charge. It is well maintained, has a Sunday School, and also provides catering and toilet facilities.

Miss Gertrude Best was a Doctor of Music and organist. She formed and trained the choir at Albion Hall. Hadwen produced a set of rules to apply to members of this group on a printed card.

> That the choir be known as the Albion Hall Choir.
> That Dr. W. R. Hadwen be President.
> That the Officers consist of Choir Leader, Secretary, Treasurer,

Auditor and Collector.

That any candidate for membership must satisfy the Choir Leader as to musical ability and general proficiency.

That any member absent from Service or Choir practice for more than two successive weeks or for four Sundays during any one quarter, failing to give satisfactory reason, ceases to be a member and must make application to the Choir Leader if desirous of re-instatement.

That every member of the Choir shall be in his or her place at 6. 20 pm on Sunday evenings.

That Choir practice be held every Tuesday evening from 8 o'clock to 9 o'clock. Punctuality is of the highest importance.

That the choice of the music to be in the hands of the President and Choir Leader and that their decision be accepted as final.

That every member pay one pence per week in order to supply funds for music, etc. This will not be expected from those unemployed.

That any person desirous of becoming Honorary Member may apply to the Choir Secretary; the fee to be not less than one shilling per annum.

That in the event of Concerts, Service of Song or other entertainment given by the Choir, every member to take part or if unable to do so, to give due notice to the Choir Leader.

That all music be the absolute property of the choir and must not be taken away without permission of the Librarian. Any music thus borrowed to be returned in good condition.

That the Annual Business Meeting be held early in March when all reports be read and Officers elected for the ensuing year.

New members shall be required to signify their assent to these rules by signing name in Register.

That the accounts be audited for presentation to the Annual Meting.

These detailed rules give some insight into the control Hadwen exhibited in his dealings at Albion Hall. He had organised the building, appointing himself as the regular evening preacher, controlling the activities of the Sunday School and choice of music of the choir etc. He left £2, 500 in his will to Dr Best in recognition of her services to the choir at Albion Hall.

Once established in Gloucester, Hadwen was an outright winner in a poll (1897) to serve on the School Board, and set about investigating the sanitary problems of the schools. He reported on conditions at Widden Street school, where the smallpox epidemic is said to have started, This resulted in the overhauling of ventilation and sanitation in the building. He monitored new building of schools closely and introduced classes in manual instruction so that skills were developed as well as 'working the brain'. He insisted that domestic science and carpentry facilities were provided. There were cases where unvaccinated children were shut out of schools and, of course, Hadwen opposed such action.

Jumping ahead a decade, it would appear that Hadwen could not pass by the idea of a project to occupy even more of his time. Gloucester traditionally had half day closing on a Thursday and this applied to the Doctor's Surgery. (This 'tradition' continued into the 1970s, some years after I joined the practice) This free time allowed Hadwen the pleasure

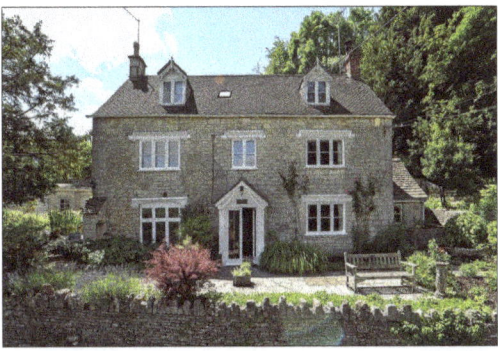

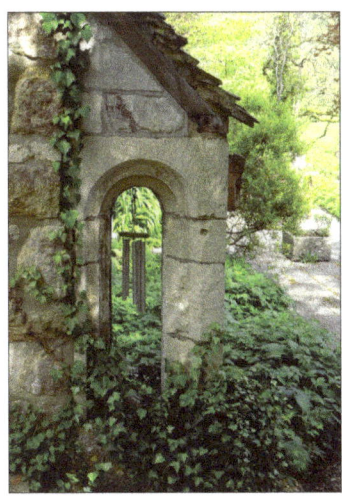

Right: 'Hillside' as it stands today
Below right: Some of the stonemasonry still incorporated into the garden.
Below: This 'arch' is almost as seen in the original black and white photograph (overleaf)

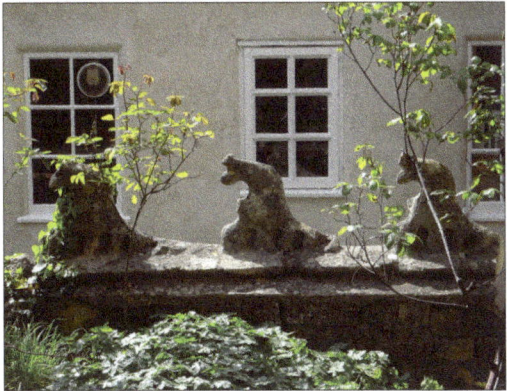

of investigating the surrounding area of Gloucester in his earlier days, on foot or bike, sometimes accompanied by his granddaughter. One afternoon while out cycling, he saw the road leading up the side of the main road to Stroud and decided to explore. This small quiet village of Pitchcombe is 7 miles from Gloucester city centre. Accordingly, in 1909, having fallen in love with the views from the village over the

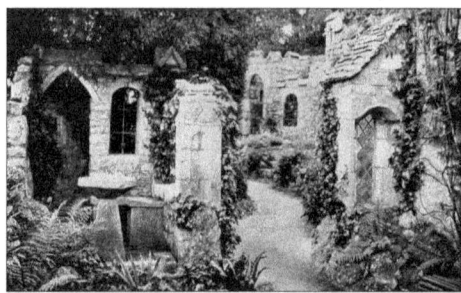
Part of the imitation ruins

Painswick valley and also the property 'Hillside' which overlooks the same scene, he proceeded immediately to negotiate the purchase of this property. It is described as an 18th-century weaver's cottage. His granddaughter describes it as his bolt-hole and hobby. He supervised the development of the garden and added recovered Cotswold stone constructed as a folly. Some of the stone may have come from the ruins of a chapel which stood nearby or as it is mentioned, from Pitchcombe Abbey. I briefly visited the property many years ago, but more recently was given a guided tour by the present owner showing me some of the original features. An old photo shows how the construction of the stones used to look. The garden has all been tastefully redesigned but some of the original stonework can easily be identified. In August 1915, he is quoted as writing ' I have finished my ruins and I am satisfied. They are as pure a bit of old-world reality as you would find, even though in a small compass'.

Hadwen's plans did not stop there. His vision was not only for himself and his wife to enjoy some relaxation but to create a 'Care Home' with nutritious food; although not stated one assumes it would be a vegetarian diet. There were six bedrooms and the doors are still numbered as such. The 'attic' is now a large studio but originally would suitably accommodate the nurse or manageress in charge. Originally a nurse was appointed but eventually a 'housekeeper' replaced her, one assumes on grounds of expense.

Hadwen sent some of his needy patients there, probably at his expense, but other guests came from all over the country. Hadwen still spent his Thursday afternoons there when he could and his wife would stay for several weeks at a time.

Eventually, after Hadwen's death, his granddaughter occupied the house for some years.

Opposite and following pages: Scans of the original pamphlet giving applicants an overview of what the 'Holiday Home' had to offer.

Cotswold Hills Food Reform Holiday Home

"Hillside," Pitchcombe, near Stroud, Glos.

THIS Establishment is conducted with a view to afford convalescents and persons requiring rest and change and country air, an opportunity for gaining strength and recuperation among the delightful attractions of the Cotswolds.

The house stands 600 feet

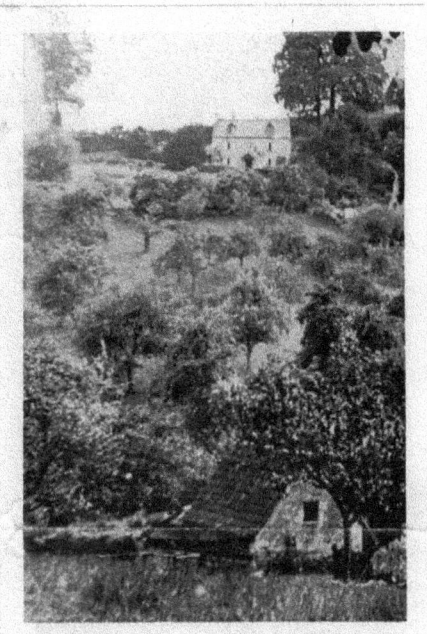

"Hillside," as seen from the Village.

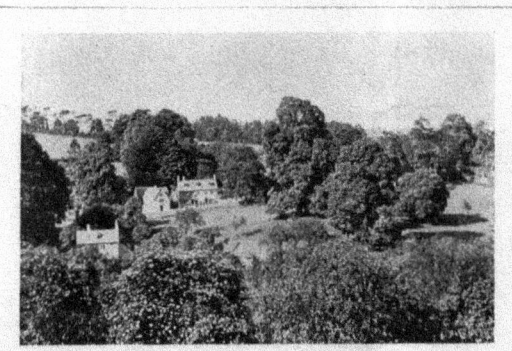

Pitchcombe—the Village as seen from "Hillside."

above sea level, and overlooks one of the loveliest valleys in the Cotswold district.

From the windows a view is obtained which it is impossible to adequately represent in any picture, where a panorama of thickly-

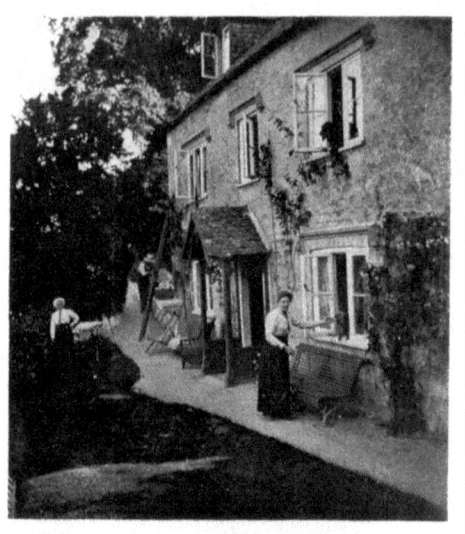

"Hillside."

wooded hills rise beyond the intervening valley, while immediately below the house lies the exquisitely situated and picturesque village of Pitchcombe. Behind, the hill still rises another 200 feet to an extensive Common, bordered by woods, which can be traversed for miles, commanding a fine view of the Golden Valley.

Town dwellers will find the quiet of "Hillside" an admirable nerve-tonic, and lovers of nature will be surprised to realize that winter or summer, wet weather or fine, makes little difference to the beauty of the landscape which constantly lies before their eyes.

There are beautiful walks in all directions, and Golf Links within short distance. There is a Motor-bus Service to Stroud, 1½ miles away, from whence there is a quick and frequent train service on the G.W.R. to London and Motor-bus to Cheltenham, 7 miles distant.

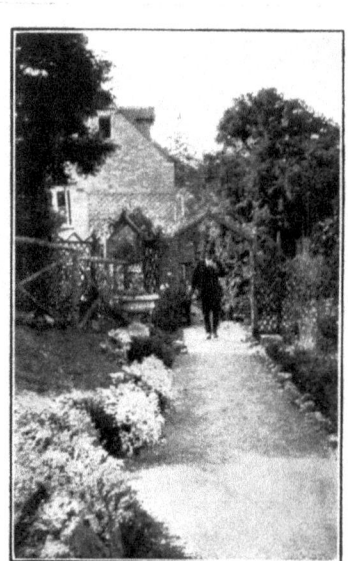

Garden Walk.

Only a small number can be accommodated at one time, the conditions being entirely those of family life, and no more are received than can be comfortably situated.

The Dietary is a food reform one, with farmhouse eggs, butter and milk.

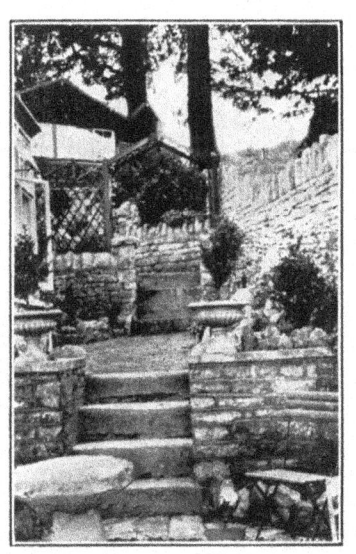

Corner of the Terrace at "Hillside."

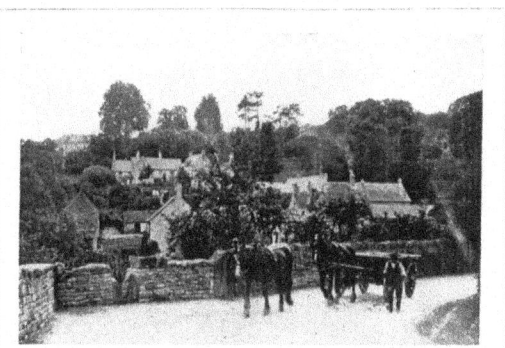

Pitchcombe Village, showing "Hillside" on summit to the left.

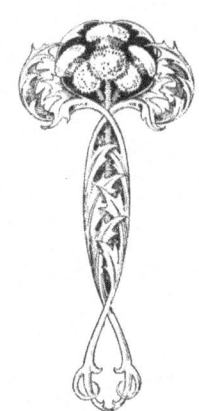

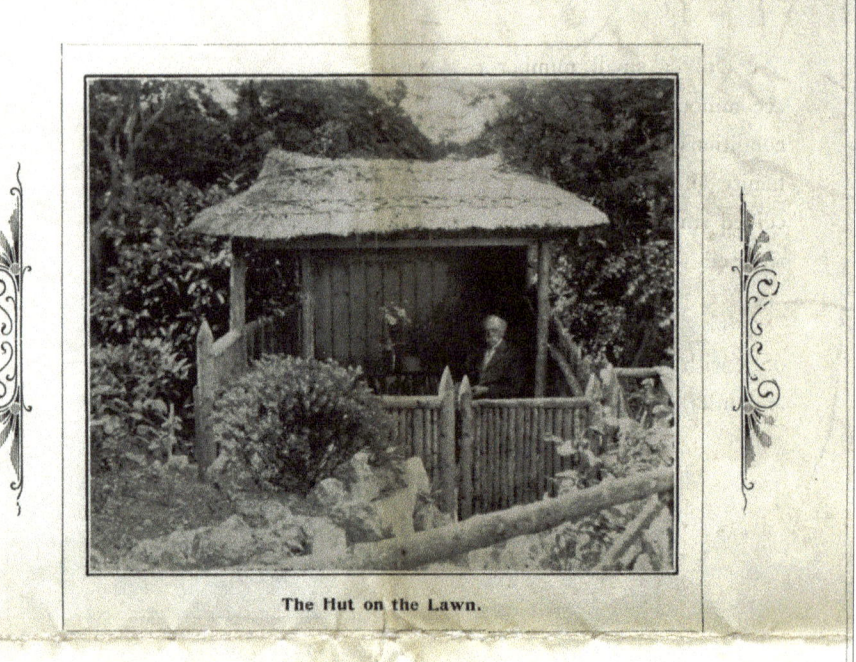

The Hut on the Lawn.

Terms for Board and Residence:

35/- ... ... per week.

Children - One Guinea per week.

There are two double-bedded rooms which if used by a single person, the terms would be Two Guineas per week.

For further particulars apply to
The Manageress,
" Hillside," Pitchcombe.
near Stroud, Glos.

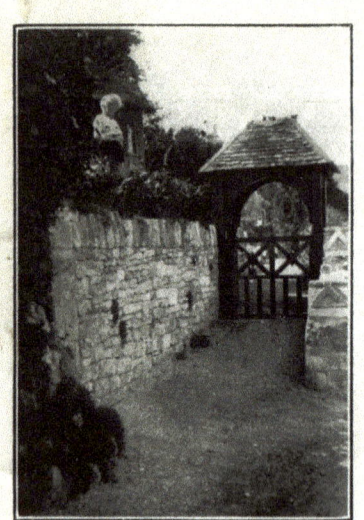

Entrance to "Hillside."

4
EXPLANATION OF CONDITIONS IN GLOUCESTER AFFECTING THE 1896 SMALLPOX OUTBREAK

THE POOR LAW Amendment Act (England & Wales), under the governance of the Poor Law Commissioners, became effective in 1834 with further updating in 1884. Urban areas elected Boards of Guardians who were responsible for Unions based on a group of Parishes. The Gloucester city urban area population was 39, 444. The boundaries of the union did not conform with those of the Parliamentary constituency. Amongst their duties and responsibilities was to look after the poor and this included the running of the workhouses. The poor rate was collected by the overseer to cover the costs which included doctor's fees, medicine, midwife and even coffins and other approved expenses. Much poor relief was given to families of men who died from infectious diseases.

The Public Health Act of 1848 was passed following a major outbreak of cholera. The improvements planned were the repair of drainage and sewers pipework, removal of all refuse, providing clean drinking water and appointing a medical officer and sanitary inspector to every town. The expense was to be financed from central loans and repaid from rates. The Act provided a framework for action but was not compulsory.

The Vaccination Acts came into force in 1853; by then variolation had become illegal and vaccination was free of charge. Children were to be vaccinated within three months of birth by a public vaccinator or medical practitioner. The procedure had to be notified to the local registrar. The fine for not complying then was £1. By 1867 the Poor-Law Guardians were to control vaccination in their Unions, the vaccinators fee incurred was one to three shillings. Arm to arm vaccination was banned. In 1871 the law appointed Vaccination Officers who could also authorise a defendant to appear in court for non compliance and by 1873 vaccination was compulsory. The approved vaccine by the Board of Guardians was to use calf-lymph, (apparently proving to be more potent and long lasting) rather than humanised lymph. This all caused considerable hostility in many towns. By 1898 a Royal Commission removed 'cumulative penalties' for opposing the procedure and safer vaccines were to be used. Anyone wanting to take advantage as a conscientious objector had to satisfy two magistrates by arguing their case. Many such officials refused or delayed such permission and by 1906 only 40, 000 exemptions were obtained. The 1907 Act allowed a statutory declaration by a parent that he believed vaccination would be prejudicial to the health of a child. Magistrates could witness the declaration.

I have been able to read the minutes of the meetings of the Poor Law Guardians in Gloucester from 1887 for the next few years. Also, I have tried to digest the 24-page report by the committee appointed by the Board or Guardians to organise and carry out the general vaccination of Gloucester city and District under the Superintendent Dr Francis D. Bond, MD. Briefly, there was much heated discussion for and against obeying the Act that made vaccination compulsory, the main issue being that it would be illegal to vote against compulsory vaccination, though some Guardians in other cities had done so. The city guardians were aware that the local population would support only a move against compulsion. Apparently the law made for compulsory re-vaccination for civil servants, postmen, soldiers and sailors but this seemed to infringe human rights. Figures were produced to show there was a health risk and even death from the procedure, quoting that out of Gloucester's population of 40, 000, 29 deaths occurred following vaccination. Other statistics showed that the best vaccinated towns had the highest rate of smallpox. Many cities had ceased prosecutions of those who refused to comply with the Act.

Worries were expressed about the purity of the lymph used and risk of transmitted disease or even hereditary problems. The Board voted against compulsory vaccination of the city population hoping that none of their members would have to go to prison! The instruction was that the vaccination officer take no further action to prosecute individuals until authorised by the Board. Further meetings and motions were debated but the general instruction was that prosecutions for non compliance of the Act should not proceed.

Apparently, the local MP, influenced by the views of the electorate, initially had a negative view on the question of compulsory vaccination. However, he later vacillated from anti to pro in Parliament. This indecision was attacked by Hadwen in the form of a skittish poem published in the *Gloucester Journal* in 1898 under the pseudonym 'Spectator' and consisted of no fewer than nineteen verses aimed at the MP's change of loyalty to his electors.

Centrally, the Local Government Board recommended revaccination every twelve years, or every ten years if there was immediate danger of smallpox. By 1888 a Medical Officer of Health and an official public vaccinator was appointed. In 1889 the local Board should form a committee to present evidence to the Royal Commission from parents who believed their children had suffered injury or death due to vaccination. They would also collect names of people who wished to present their views to the Commission on either side of the vaccination question. The Board itself should not express an opinion until the Commission reported.

In 1891 a gentleman offered to supply, gratuitously, calf-lymph to the Public Vaccinator but the Board decided against this offer.

In November 1895, The new Medical Officer of Health reported to the Board that there were eight cases of smallpox in the isolation hospital. By January 1896 there were 36 cases, and he stated vaccination and revaccination must be encouraged, however no specific action was taken. The Board of Guardians and local authority were charged with failing to enforce the law by Mr Justice Grantham. The Jenner Society was formed to produce publicity documents and notices to counteract similar advertising literature printed by the anti-vaccination campaigners.

A meeting of all members of the medical profession in the city was convened, probably coerced by the BMA, and they apparently excluded Hadwen from their deliberations, he becoming a 'social outlaw'. They proposed an increase in hospital accommodation for infectious disease cases both for the present and future, assessing efficacy of vaccination long-term, and persuading the Guardians to comply with the Order of the Local Government Board and prepare a list of unvaccinated children.

By March 1896 more public vaccinators and district nurses were appointed, but still by May it was estimated that there were 3, 000 unvaccinated children in the city.

All too late, a grant of £4,000 was made by the Local Government Board for improvements in drinking water and sewerage facilities.

It is of interest that no mention is made in the minutes of the Board of Guardians of the influence of Dr Hadwen on the views of the local population.

Most importantly, the situation in the city was described by Dr Hadwen before he moved to Gloucester. His visits (including home visits) and inspection of the city facilities resulted in the following detailed and important letter to the *Bristol Mercury* newspaper:

THE OUTBREAK OF SMALLPOX IN GLOUCESTER AND ITS CAUSES
Challenge from a Doctor to a Doctor
April 30th, 1896
National Anti-Vaccination League, 50, Parliament Street London SW

The objects of this league is to repeal the Vaccination Acts, the disestablishment and disendowment of the practice of Vaccination, and the abolition of all regulations in regard to vaccination as conditions of employment in State Departments or of admission to Educational or other Institutions.

Every opponent of Compulsory Vaccination in the UK is earnestly invited to join and co-operate with the League.

To the Editor of the Bristol Mercury.
Sir, I have drawn attention in your columns to the sanitary conditions of Gloucester. I have declared my conviction that it is not the unvaccinated element in the community, but the insanitary conditions existing prior to the outbreak and gradual growth of smallpox from 1893, which furnish the explanation why the epidemic has so fastened itself upon the Southern portion of the city.

Dr Bond, Medical Officer of Health for the rural district of Gloucester, has declared my statements to be 'ludicrously in-accurate' and I have offered, in reply, to forfeit £50 to the Gloucester Smallpox Hospital if he can disprove them. He, having publicly challenged my statements, now wishes me to state what it is that he has challenged! It is obviously for him to do this, but my case is so clear that I will summarise it thus:-

Propositions
A That Gloucester be divided into two halves by a line drawn east and

west through St. Michael's Square, both halves, North and South, were equally unvaccinated.

B That the epidemic has been practically confined to the South Gloucester.

C That some causes outside vaccination must therefore be sought to account for the prevalence of smallpox in this particular portion of the city.

D That the insanitary conditions in South Gloucester were such as to fully account for the localisation of the epidemic in it.

Evidence

1 Gloucester has suffered for years from a shortage of water supply.

2 The city supply, by great vigilance and economy and repeated warnings from the authorities, had been reduced to a dangerous limit.

3 The Citizens have had to resort to the Canal and River (into which the sewerage of the city empties) when their ordinary supplies ran short.

4 The necessity in 1893 and 1894 was signalised by a large increase of typhoid fever, no fewer than 49 cases being attributed by the Medical Officer of Health to this cause in 1884.

5 For years past, hundreds of houses in the city have rain water supply from the dangerous shallow wells, liable to serious contamination by constant leakage into them from house drains, a great many lying in the district where smallpox commenced.

6 Many houses, mainly at the South-West corner, where smallpox has been very severe, have been supplied with Lyson's or Hempstead water, which is not only unsafe to use, but has not pressure enough to drive it into the flush boxes.

7 As late as to the end of 1894 (during which seven cases of smallpox appeared in the city) there were still 141 houses using shallow well water, 155 houses using Lyson's water, and 190 houses which, supplied by city water, were not supplied by flushing boxes.

8 The supply of water was insufficient without copious rains to flush the closets, house drainage and the sewers effectively.

9 The prolonged frosts of the winter 1894-95 followed by the prolonged summer's drought, a phenomenal absence of rain in the fall of the year and at the beginning of this year, served to intensify the normal condition of things in the city. In the added districts of south Gloucester, inhabited for the most part by a large working class population, with water pipes long frozen, the house drains clogged for weeks, (in many

cases reported defective), and no subsequent rain storms to flush either them or the sewers. This resulted in foul gasses generated having to find an exit either through the sink traps and w. c. 's or the sewer manholes in the streets. The pent up conditions of the poorest class, the families of casual labourers etc, dreading to open door or window for the cold, with insufficient firing to promote ventilation, dependent on charity for bare food and clothing, such conditions were specially conducive to low vitality and susceptibility to disease.

10 Flushing of sewers has been sparingly performed owing to shortage of water until recent weeks. Vigorous action in this respect has only been since the epidemic has fairly got abroad.

11 The awful stench of sewer gas arising from many of the street manholes has become a byword in the city, and the contiguity of some of them to smallpox stricken houses is highly suggestive. Plugging the holes with wooden stoppers and covering them in other ways has had to be resorted to, but it has been officially stated it would be a dangerous experiment to stop them altogether, as it would force sewer gas into the houses instead of, as now, into the open air. As far back as 1881 the Medical Officer reported concerning an epidemic of scarlet fever then raging throughout the smallpox area: 'The constant escape of sewer gas in the streets where children are passing and playing, must tend to produce an injurious effect on the health of such children, and consequently have rendered them more susceptible of receiving infection, and less able to combat successfully with the disease when infected'

12 During the cholera scare in the latter part of 1892-93 three extra sanitary inspectors were temporarily appointed to make a house to house inspection, and a terrible condition of things was discovered. 'Houses without proper water supply, closets without flush boxes, indoor soil pipes (often leaking) house drains (very imperfect) going under the houses with only protection of such water seal as exists in the ordinary useless traps, and closets not ventilated'. During 1893 (when smallpox first put in an appearance) further investigation discovered no less than 3648 similar sanitary defects. That fresh discoveries were made in 1894 (when the number of smallpox cases had more than doubled) is clear from the admission of the Medical Officer of Health to the Board of Guardians on January 28th, 1896, that 'during the past two years' 1894 and 1895 (in the last year smallpox cases had quadrupled those of 1894) they had had to remedy no fewer than 3541 sanitary defects.

13 Judging by non-official information supplied to me from various

quarters, numerous defects of a similar nature still existed when in 1896 the gradually growing storm burst with all its fury upon South Gloucester, and still exists at the present time.

14 Zymotic diseases have been prevalent and have found a home principally in South Gloucester to which smallpox has been practically restricted. Measles in 1892 and 1893 assumed a severe type, and in the latter year 36 deaths occurred therefrom. Scarlet fever reached 360 cases in 1892, and 107 cases in 1894. Diphtheria, which has been a fairly constant visitor, and had been raging throughout 1891, was epidemic in 1892, the cases numbering 136, not one of which could be isolated, as the hospital was full of scarlet fever patients; 59 cases occurred in 1893 and 33 cases in 1894. This disease has again been reported recently in its old haunts in South Gloucester. Speaking of diphtheria in 1893, the Medical Officer of Health for the city of Gloucester remarks 'I think little doubt can be entertained as to the connection between this disease and the unhealthy surroundings. Damp walls, damp cellars, defective house drains, imperfect ventilation and the like are generally found where it is prevalent, and during the year just past we have found most of these conditions where diphtheria made anything of a stand'.

15 Complaints have been made about the overcrowding of the Board schools for the past years, a condition rendering children highly susceptible to Zymotic disease. The grant of £841 was withheld in 1894 for three months owing to this condition of things, and the threat of a heavy fine by the Education Department was made in 1895, unless extra accommodation was speedily provided. Widden Street Infant School (at the back of Barton Street), under the same roof as the boys and girls rooms, which were greatly overcrowded, was the first infant's school attacked by the smallpox. Until then the unvaccinated children of Gloucester had suffered but little, the disease having commenced with and had been largely confined to vaccinated persons of older years. Forty five children in this school were suddenly infected. The first to be attacked was a vaccinated teacher. The sanitary arrangements in connection with this infant's school were such that the Board contemplated spending £100 to £150 upon them.

16 The next infants' school to be attacked was St. Luke's, (New Street- now St Paul's) where 31 children were suddenly infected. The maximum number of children allowed in a school by a Government is 224 or 225. The average attendance for the past year, according to the vicar, was 218 which leaves 6 or 7 short of the full allowance, as the Rev. H. Proctor

states that 'the attendance of infants is always worst in the winter months' and that 'the attendance at the time of the outbreak was much less' than the average (only 93), it proves conclusively that, during the summer which preceded the winter's smallpox outbreak in the school, it must have been in a congested condition, and the constitutions of the children, to say the least of it, had not been fortified against the coming epidemic storm. *The Times* of 3rd inst. , p. 10, writing on the report of the Poor Law Schools Committee, points out that 'besides causing the spread of the disease, the aggregation of children affects their health, by lowering their vitality, and diminishing their nervous energy. '

17 The inadequacy of hospital accommodation to see the requirements of the approaching epidemic, of which warning was not wanting, for 3 previous years, is another serious blot upon city administration. In 1892, under stress of the extensive epidemic of scarlet fever, the hospital accommodation, which until then provided but 16 beds, was quickly trebled under the plea of declared 'urgency' thus providing accommodation even then for only 48 cases. An extra block, further removed from the others, for smallpox, was urged in vain, even though the following year the attention of the Sanitary Authority was officially drawn to the fact that smallpox was busy in various places around them. In the first and last clauses of the medical manifesto in January last, signed by 22 doctors, attention was again drawn to the inadequacy of hospital accommodation. Then came the sudden outbreak in Widden Street and St. Luke's infant schools. London and Provincial papers were immediately flooded with sensational and panic-stricken letters (like that of Dr Davies of Bristol), telling the story of the sickening sight of which those poor little suffering and dying victims presented in the pestiferous atmosphere of the overcrowded and undermanned hospital wards, where they had been taken at night from their mothers and their homes, and congregated together under the plea of 'isolation'. The terrible responsibility which lay upon the shoulders of the city Council in not having provided the first line of defence was shifted on to that of the Guardians, who had wisely refused to enforce the Vaccination Act, and upon the parents who had declined to comply with it. In the worked-up panic which has ensued it has been sought by every possible means to divert the attention of the public from the real causes which have favoured the spread of smallpox, and to absorb it with the despairing and superstitious cry of 'Vaccination!'.

18 I conclude with the health protest of Mr Edwin Chadwick, the

veteran sanitarian, who said 'Smallpox, typhus and other fevers occur in common conditions of foul air, stagnant putrefaction, bad house drainage, sewers of deposit, excrement in sodden sites, filthy street surfaces, impure water and overcrowding. The entire removal of such conditions is the only effectual prevention of diseases of those species, whether ordinary or extraordinary visitations'.

I have now told the other side of the story. Dr Bond has only to deny the truth of my propositions, and to state that he accepts my challenge, and will, as evidence of good faith, agree to forfeit his £50 in the event of his failure to disprove them, then the preliminaries for the adjudication of the matter can be proceeded with.

I am, Sir, your obedient servant, Walter R Hadwen, LRCP MRCS, etc Highbridge, Somerset, April 28th, 1896.

P. S. - In the recently published vital statistics of the city of Gloucester, for the quarter ending March 31st, 1896, striking corroboration is afforded of the fact that smallpox has been practically confined to the one insanitary quarter of the city I have drawn attention to, for the whole of the 146 deaths from that disease during this period are recorded as occurring in the South Hamlet, in which district 156 of the 159 deaths from zygotic disease took place.

The Medical Officer of Health reported to the Gloucester Sanitary Authority, on 30th March, 1894, respecting the water supply mentioned in paragraph 6, as follows;- 'a year or two ago Mr Read (the city surveyor) and myself made a systematic inspection of this system of supply, and we found that, from its source to its delivery, this water received large quantities of sewerage and the pollution'.

(from the *TRUTH* April 30th 1896)
'Here is a matter which seems well serving of notice in connection with the smallpox epidemic in Gloucester. In May of last year a gentleman who was doing clerical duty in the town found a case of smallpox in his district and also that every attempt was being made to conceal the fact. In the course of his visitations he also formed the opinion that the sanitary considerations of parts of the town were most defective and dangerous, hundreds of houses being without either water or a drainage system, and entirely dependent upon well water, which was of the most unsatisfactory quality. Not having, I presume, much confidence in the local authorities, this gentleman, later in the year, reported the result

FOUR REASONS
WHY YOU SHOULD NOT HAVE YOUR CHILDREN VACCINATED.

1.—Vaccination affords no protection against Small Pox.
In Birmingham, in 1874, over 600 persons, mostly vaccinated, died of Small Pox, although the Public Vaccinator received, in 1873, in fees and awards for his *successful* vaccinations, £1,173!

2.—It so lowers the vitality that they are renderd more liable to other diseases.
Notice the great increase of Measles, Whooping-cough, and Scarlatina since Vaccination has been compulsory.

3.—Great risk is incurred of contaminating their blood with loathsome, and incurable maladies. In 1872-73-74, 1,074 Infants and Children, under five years of age, died of Syphilis in London alone. From these probably thousands were vaccinated, **and contaminated.**
See Essays on Vaccination by Dr. Pearce, Dr. Collins, and others; also evidence of the eminent Surgeon, J. Hutchinson, Esq., in the *Medical Times and Gazette*, Feb. 1st and 8th, 1873, for revolting revelations on this point.

4.—Death from Pyæmia or Erysipelas often follows the operation: 139 children under five years of age, died in London of Erysipelas in 1874.

Be not deceived! Think for yourself! The insertion of corrupt, diseased matter (falsely called Vaccine Lymph) into the blood of healthy infants, can produce nothing but its legitimate fruit—Corruption—Disease—and Death.
The country will never be rid of Small Pox until Vaccination is prohibited.

Published by the Society for Suppressing Compulsory Vaccination.
W. YOUNG, *Hon. Sec.*, 8, Neeld Terrace, Harrow Road, W.

January, 1876.

PLEASE POST THIS AT ONCE.

Vaccination Acts, 1867=1907.

To Mr. W. F. Field.

It is *not* my intention to * *have my child vaccinated—I have a conscientious objection to Child murder*

* Here state if you are having the child vaccinated by Public Vaccinator or your private Doctor. If by the Public Vaccinator, say when you would like him to call.

Signed *H C A Digby*

Address *18 Bensor Road, Twickenham*

Date as post mark.

Anti-vaccination Campaign-advice and exemption form for the parent to sign, confirming their intention not to have their child vaccinated. Dr Hadwen as a JP, offered to witness such declarations without charge.

of his observations to the Local Government Board, but at the same time requested that his name might not be mentioned in connection with the matter- a very natural and reasonable request, far as I can see. He received the following official reply:- "The president of the Local Government Board cannot take cognisance of any common actions of this nature without permission to reveal the name of the person giving the communication to the district and local authorities. ' In any case, the rule here laid down would seem to me a foolish manifestation of red tape. It is easy to imagine potent reasons which would lead to the person giving the information to the Local Government Board not to desire to appear publicly in the locality in support of his statements; and, one would think that the Local Government Board, in the public interest, make a point of at least ascertaining its accuracy. In the present instance there is every reason to suppose that if the Board had taken the hint thus conveyed to them, the disastrous epidemic at Gloucester might have been nipped in the bud. The information was not sent anonymously, but came from a gentleman in a responsible position, whose faith there was not the slightest reason to doubt, and by the expenditure of a few shillings on enquiries, the Local Government Board could have discovered last Autumn that there had been smallpox in the town, that the local authority had attempted to hush the matter up. and that the sanitary condition of at least a quarter of the town were such that an outbreak of smallpox there would be like dropping a lighted match into a powder-magazine. If it does nothing else, the outbreak in Gloucester ought to teach the Local Government Board a little wisdom.

Not only was this letter published in the *Bristol Mercury* but also reproduced as a pocket sized booklet of sixteen pages reprinted by the National Anti-Vaccination League in London, and so Hadwen's assessment of the situation in Gloucester was spread country wide for all to read.

Hadwen decried the work of Pasteur and Koch and also Metchikoff's theory of phagocytes mopping up microbes and debris in the blood. Miasma is the theory of noxious bad air or night air resulting from rotting organic matter and thus disease was spread. Miasma, as such, does not seem to be mentioned in any of Hadwen's writings but his whole philosophy on promoting good health revolved around improved sanitation and good quality drinking water, as well as reducing overcrowding and poor social conditions. He mentions 'infectious disease' and uses the general word for contagious diseases, 'Zymotic Disease' but gives no further explanation for the cause except for 'a chemical in the air'.

Hadwen was supported in his views by having the sympathy of the then proprietor of the *Citizen* local newspaper who was himself an anti-vaccinationist. However this support was undermined later by the news which stated that this man eventually undertook vaccination

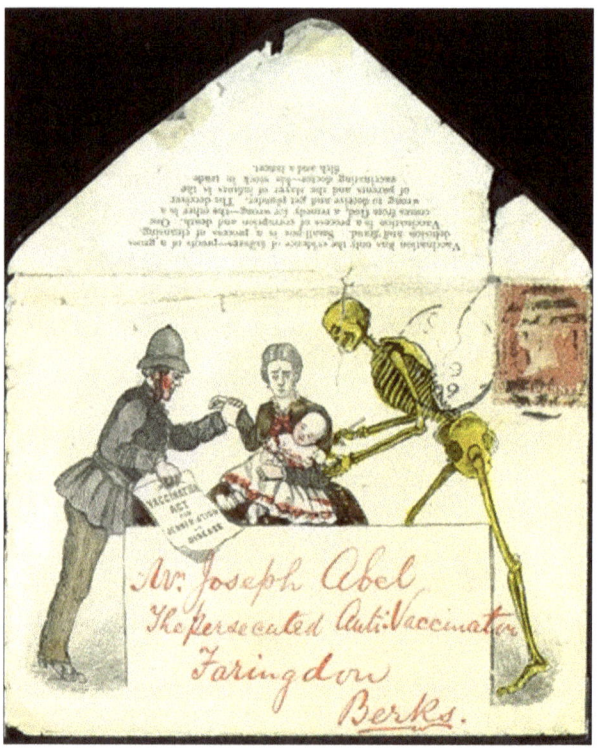

Example of more extreme publicity against vaccination

Printed on the seal flap

*'Vaccination has only the evidence of failures-proofs of a gross
delusion and fraud. Smallpox is a process of cleansing. Vaccination is a process of corruption and death. One comes from God, a remedy for wrong-the other is a wrong to deceive and get plunder. The deceiver of parents and the slayer of infants is the vaccinating doctor - his stock in trade filth and a lancet.*

owing to pressure brought to bear on him by partners and tradesmen in the city. Another false challenge was made against Hadwen that he had secretly gone to Cheltenham and been vaccinated.

On the other hand, he was at loggerheads with the Medical Officer of Health, Dr John Campbell, whom he hounded for information and statistics. The accusation was that published observations were biased or prejudiced by self-opinion or entirely inaccurate. Hadwen, on one of his visits to the isolation hospital, persuaded Dr. Campbell to delete the labelling 'unvaccinated' on patients' bed charts who swore they had been vaccinated. Hadwen demonstrated that old vaccination marks were covered by recent pox scabs, apparent evidence that vaccination did not protect as claimed. Hadwen was also highly critical of the claims made in the Dr. Coupland's report on the 1895-96 epidemic published in late November 1897, that was after the Royal Commission issued its final report! Figures were produced to prove that vaccination and revaccination gave protection but Hadwen produced equal facts and figures which, in his view, refuted the effectiveness of the vaccination process. Hadwen carefully dissected the evidence in the report by researching accurately and interviewing individual and family cases and their vaccination history originally in this report.

In one document, it is inferred that employees were persuaded by their employers to be vaccinated against their will and went to great lengths to counteract the procedure. They tried to neutralise the vaccinated area by 'sucking their arms as soon as they conveniently could. Others washed the incision or rubbed ointment or other applications on the wound; others poulticed it. In fact they did their best, so far as their own ingenuity, or the suggestion of other malcontents like themselves, enabled them, to defeat the work of the vaccinator'. These manoeuvres may have been partially successful!

However, Gloucester's reputation as a city was stigmatised and advice was publicised 'Do not travel to Gloucester'. Politically, the Labour Party in 1900 contained a commitment to 'No compulsory vaccination' in their General Election Manifesto.

5
FURTHER CHALLENGES

Locally, Hadwen was soon elected on to the Sanitary Committee. He helped to action the improvements in drainage and sewer development in the city. Sanitary matters were Hadwen's passion.

In 1898, having satisfied the residency qualification, he was elected to the city Council representing Barton Ward and resigned in 1904. There was debate in Council over the plan to inaugurate electric trams to replace horse drawn vehicles. This plan was opposed by Hadwen, he having thoroughly researched similar ventures entered upon by other cities throughout the country. All the detail was noted on profitability, mainly a loss, and apparently he warned that certain gradients would defeat the trams traction. Ultimately the tracks were taken up and motor-omnibuses substituted. His predictions were correct.

He argued that the cruel exposure of cattle to the heat in the market place (now King's Square) was unacceptable. A fine avenue of plane-trees were planted to give shade (1920)

The most notable appointment for Hadwen was as a city Magistrate in 1909. His court day was a Friday and his reputation was one of leniency. His position as a magistrate had repercussions later in the story of his life.

The next major step in Hadwen's public life was eventually to have national implications.

William Tebb FRGS, was a wealthy vegetarian, teetotaller and anti-vivisectionist as well as anti-vaccinationist. He involved himself in many causes including the abolition of slavery. He describes himself as 'Corresponding Member of the Royal Academy of Medical Sciences, Palermo' whatever that might mean! I have mentioned his name in Chapter 2. In 1895 he was the main author of the book *Premature Burial and how it may be prevented*. The editor was Dr Edward Perry Vollum, M. D. , an ex-USA Army Colonel who died in 1902. In 1904

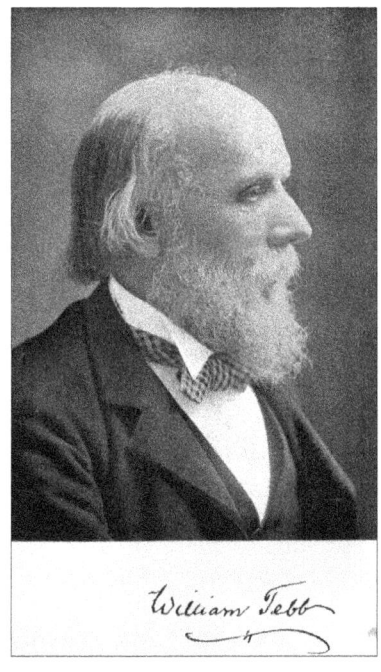

William Tebb FRGS

Tebb invited Hadwen to be the new editor of the second edition, reducing some of the original content and adding new material. The subject was of great interest, particularly in the Victorian era, and the book reveals the need that 'Parliament ensure that no medical certificate be accepted unless the person signing it shall have seen and carefully examined the body of the person so certified etc'. I have attempted to summarise the content of this quite comprehensive book and this can be found in the Appendices. This must have occupied a considerable amount of time and effort by Hadwen.

Vivisection in England and medical laboratory experiments were not as developed as on the Continent. By the 1870s the activities of British physiologists and their animal experiments were becoming common knowledge and this provoked the anti-vivisection movement to gain recognition and support.

Frances Power Cobbe, born in Dublin in 1822, played a major role over 40 years, in the anti-vivisection cause, which was a passion until her dying day. Eventually the campaigning resulted in the formation of the British Union Against Vivisection (BUAV) in 1898 which wanted 'abolition' not just a law to control laboratory conditions. Her aim was to reduce animal suffering which she considered a moral issue. Cobbe was elected President at a public meeting in Bristol. The Union Journal was the *Abolitionist*. Cobbe, herself, was not a vegetarian.

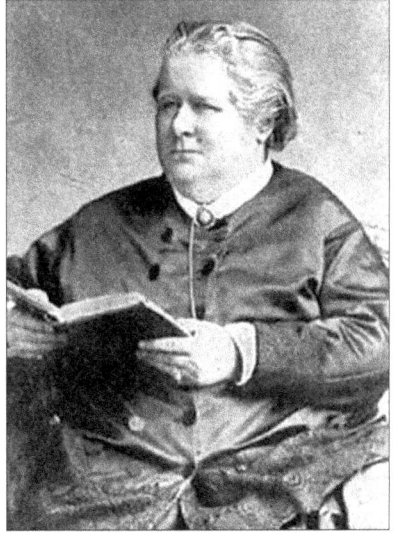

Francis Power Cobbe

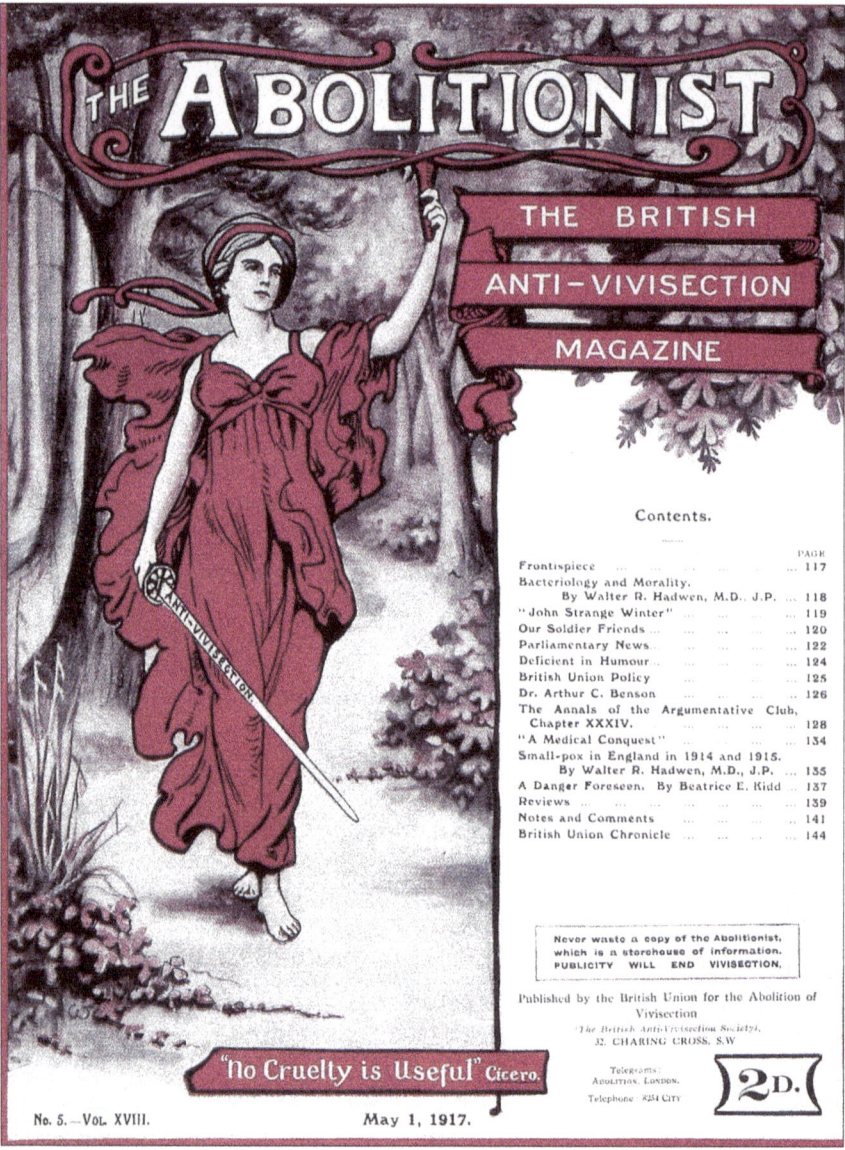

The Animal Protection Act was aimed at preventing harm and suffering to horses and cattle. A Royal Commission reported in 1876 and after modifications received assent but it had no 'teeth' to abolish vivisection. It took 110 years, until the Animals (Scientific Procedures) Act of 1986, for attitudes to alter. Cobbe, looking to the future and a successor, sent a 'spy' to Gloucester to get a first-hand assessment of Hadwen and his views and activities. He was invited to join the Union and immediately began to speak at meetings and contributed articles to the *Abolitionist* which first was published in 1899 and produced monthly thereafter. The editor appointed at that time subsequently died, Hadwen became the anonymous and unpaid editor of the journal for the next 20 years.

In the United States a new major outbreak of smallpox occurred in the 1870s as a result of vaccination procedures declining in the population and therefore susceptibility was increased. Due to many of the States trying to impose and enforce vaccination by law there was a reaction and resistance in many communities. In 1879 William Tebb visited the United States as leading British anti-vaccinationist and anti-vivisectionist, and this resulted in the founding of various state Anti-vaccination Leagues. Ultimately, after many political battles and riots, the compulsory vaccination laws were repealed.

Cobbe died in 1904, aged 81 years and Hadwen was summoned to Llanelltyd in Wales. He was requested to attend Cobbe at her residence, Hengwrt. This was her express wish, found in a telegram at her bedside. He was to perform upon her body the operation of severing an artery in order to ensure she was really dead, reflecting people's fear of Premature Burial. Her will was contested in a drawn-out legal process concerning her substantial donation to the Union of £4, 500. It was only by 1907 that this problem was resolved, but to keep BUAV afloat Hadwen subsidised with a small loan. Her death was reported in all the national newspapers and the *BMJ* paid tribute to her.

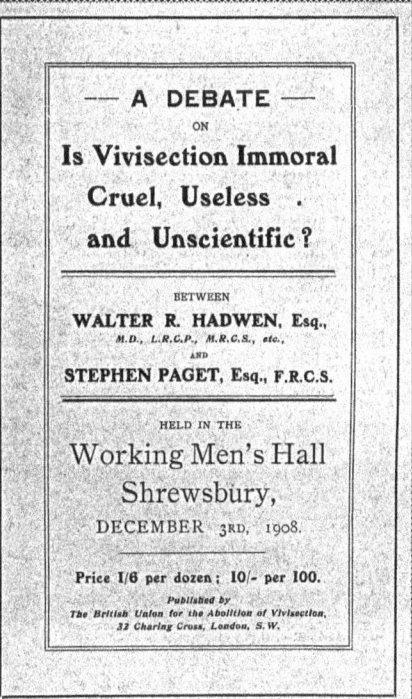

By 1904, documents show that Beatrice Kidd, co-author of Hadwen's biography, became Hadwen's contact in London and also in her position as BUAV secretary. She claims she received a letter from Hadwen virtually every day. Her initial involvement in the antivivisection movement was to work in a propagandist shop in Llangollen! At the London Office she organised debating classes each month to encourage

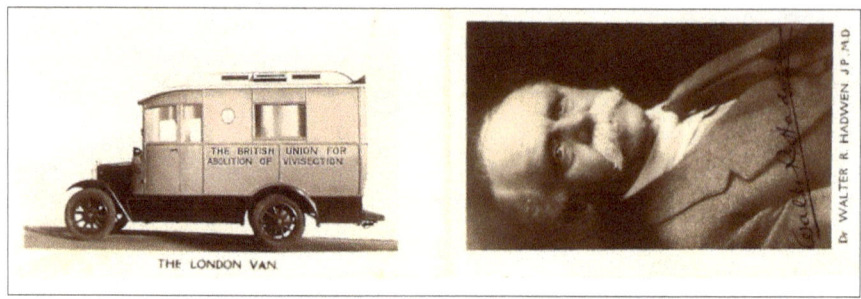

*Folding gloss photo print monthly Calendar card printed for 1929-
The first anti-vivisection van was made available from 1924*

the study of the Union's literature and how to answer opponents' questions. Instruction was given on the legal, historical and medical aspects of vivisection. Hadwen continued his support for BUAV and was elected President in 1910.

The anti-vaccination League and the anti-vivisection Union shared ideals to a certain extent. Both had offices in London, the address varying on documents The BUAV main address in 1905 was 32 Charing Cross Road. It seems that, in the end, both organisations shared premises at 47, Whitehall, London. An earlier address was Upper Charing Cross Road which was later incorporated into Whitehall.

BUAV's aim was 'To keep unalterably before its members and the public the fundamental principle of their warfare with scientific cruelty, namely, that it is a great Sin-which can only be opposed absolutely, and without attempts at delusive compromises of any kind. ' The Union argued that there was cruelty in vivisection whether anaesthetic was used or not. They claimed that vivisection was an unscientific practice and results of animal experiments were both unreliable and could not be extrapolated to humans.

In July 1905 Hadwen attended the Annual Meeting of BUAV at Caxton Hall in London expressing his views. To quote: 'The entire system of vivisection is a veritable fountain of immorality and a delusion' and 'it is God-like to protect those who cannot protect themselves' and 'a great duty in life is not to give pain'. Again he argued for total abolition of vivisection. Campaigning started with the use of shops, on short term leases in prime spots, to display leaflets, publications and posters to which there was a very positive reaction from the public. Hadwen travelled to Wrexham to speak to an audience of 1, 000 where the BUAV shop was very active. Women played a major part in the Union as this gave them an entry into public life, which was recognised by the Union and their efforts ensured the success of the cause. Women volunteers were known as ' Band of Service' working as sandwich-board advertisers and fundraisers.

By 1912 the Union had 49 branches, opening new offices in Manchester to spread their campaign in the North, and eventually Scotland also was affiliated to the Union. A campaign shop was opened in Edinburgh where the medical school had the reputation as a 'great vivisector centre'. In 1912 the shop was stormed by medical students, 26 of whom were arrested and fined. Grace Hadwen and Nurse Cross, a Union organiser, were in the shop at the time. The *Abolitionist* increased its content from eight to twenty pages; it could not exceed 24 pages because of the weight limit of a one penny postage! Distribution was enhanced by the copy being for sale at W. H. Smith. By 1914 public meetings totalled 260. The Annual public meeting was initially held at Caxton Hall but limited capacity meant a move, later, to the Grand Hall, Kensington Town Hall.

George Bernard Shaw, the playwright, addressed several of these meetings, another character of wit and eloquence. He had supported Cobbe in her earliest campaigns. Hadwen was asked by the *Standard* newspaper to write a series of three articles stating the case against vivisection. He was opposed by Stephen Paget in 1911. Paget was the founder of the Research Defence Society. A pamphlet of the debate was reproduced, its content reported in the *Cheltenham Examiner*.

Also in that year, the Government published their National Insurance Bill, primarily to protect workers against unemployment, sickness and disability but it included medical research monies of £62,500,

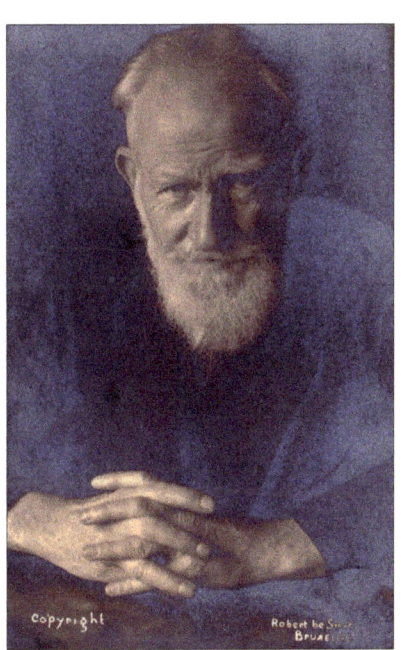

GBS in blue gown 1932

ring-fenced, which was interpreted as indirectly supporting vivisection and animal experimentation. BUAV organised a demonstration in the October which took the form of a procession from Embankment to Hyde Park, banners were on display in the distinctive red and white

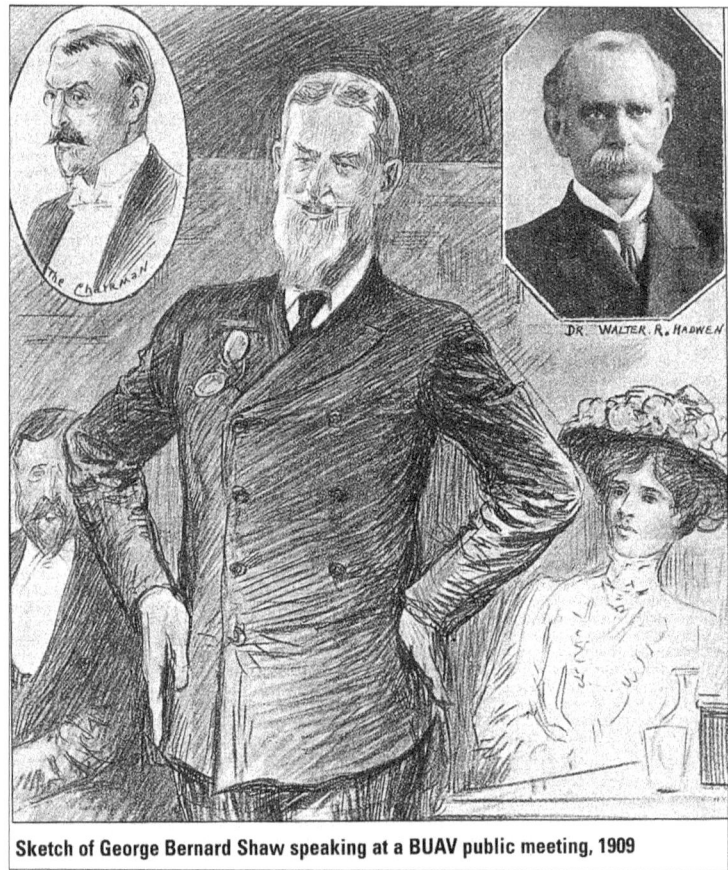

Sketch of George Bernard Shaw speaking at a BUAV public meeting, 1909

GBS alongside Hadwen

colours adopted by the Union. The highlight of the procession was a decorated carriage bearing a bust of Queen Victoria who had declared vivisection was a 'disgrace to Christianity and Humanity'. Despite this demonstration and a petition, the Bill was passed.

The year 1906 had seen the second Royal Commission on vivisection appointed but the Union had no confidence in the commission and its constitution and proceedings had to be held in secret. Hadwen's nomination to sit on the commission was rejected and the BUAV resolved not to submit evidence. The proceedings were published in a lengthy document that the common man could neither afford to purchase nor understand. George Bernard Shaw digested the contents of the report and this stimulated him to write his play ' A Doctor's Dilemma' in 1906 which brought publicity and debate on the subject of vivisection. Shaw was a vegetarian and was opposed to cruelty of any kind and supported the anti-vivisectionist movement by addressing meetings in its support and sharing a platform with Hadwen more than once. In 1913 the Medical Research Council was established to advise how the money set aside for research should be allocated, but again this was a challenge as the money was to be raised through taxpayers contribution which would compel anti-vivisectionists to pay for a practice which violated their consciences.

Mr. Chancellor MP, a BUAV supporter, set up an all-party Parliamentary anti-vivisection Committee of 50 MPs to oversee and support the interests of the anti-vivisectionist movement. At elections (two in 1910) there was an opportunity to raise the anti-vivisection views into the political arena. The Union canvassed that voters should question candidates closely and only vote for those who would support the BUAV cause. The Union hoped that Hadwen would stand as a candidate in an election but he declined. In 1911 Mr Chancellor was elected as the Parliamentary Representative of the Union and he was able to raise the topic at every opportunity. BUAV continued to preach the total abolition of vivisection and every three years the World League Against Vivisection convened. So in 1909 Hadwen was sent as a delegate to London. He debated an amendment to the rules to read 'It was open to societies and

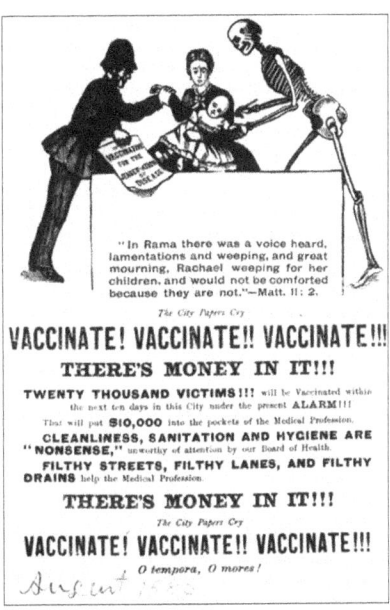

Example of typical advertising poster for Auction Sale to raise funds for those fighting against compulsory vaccination.
This poster probably pre-dates the official formation of the BUAV.

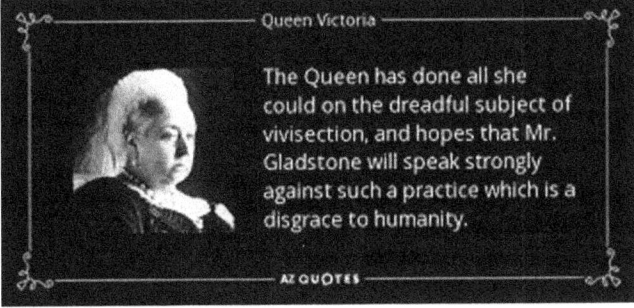

individuals in favour of total abolition of vivisection and its prohibition in law without attempts to compromise of any kind'. This was carried.

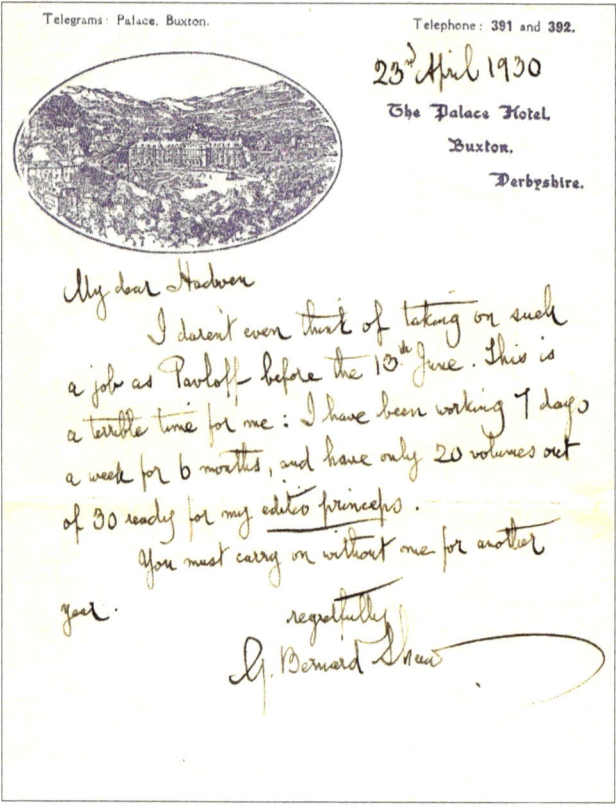

Palace Hotel, Buxton, Derbyshire 23rd April 1930

My Dear Hadwen,

I daren't even think of taking on such a job as Pavloff before the 10th of June. This is a terrible time for me: I have been working 7days a week for 6 months and have only 20 volumes out of 90 ready for my editio princeps. You must carry on without me for another year.

Regretfully,

GBS

Wording from card from Venice dated 7th April 1931 Grand Hotel, to Dr Walter Hadwen, Brunswick House, Gloucester Inglitterre

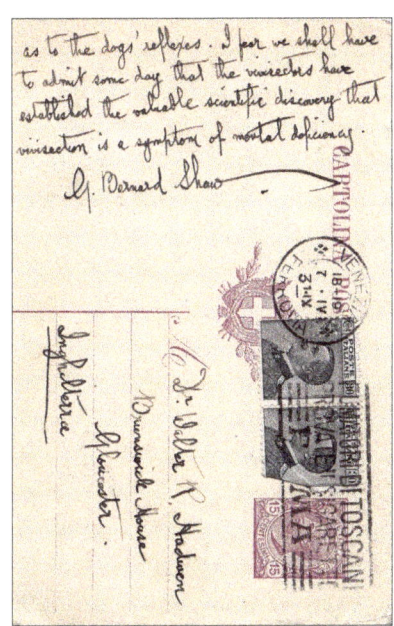

I shall not open my mouth again on the subject until I have made a careful study of that book by Pavloff of Reflexes, which is slipping into European fame as the latest Bible of Science. Pavloff persuaded H. G. Wells that his experiments were painless and that his dogs loved him, and got a testimonial from him to that effect. I have the book: and very cursory examination of it showed me that the experiments were very distressing: but it is the results that I must examine (if I can find time) as they struck me as being more instructive as to Pavloff's reasoning powers than as to the dogs' reflexes. I fear we shall have to admit some day that the vivisectors have established the valuable scientific discovery that vivisection is a symptom of mortal deficiency. GBS.

Ayot, St Lawrence, Welwyn, Herts 1932.

My Dear Hadwen,

I was in South Africa so far into the year that your letter of the 14th April has only just come to the top of the mountain of correspondence that accumulated-just too late for the meeting. You must slaughter Keith in the Abolitionist. And that £200,000! Talk of gangsters! Al Capone would have blushed.

GBS

Ayot St Lawrence. Welwyn. Herts 27/6/32

My dear Hadwen

I was in South Africa so far into the year that your letter of the 14th April has only just come to the top of the mountain of correspondence that accumulated — just too late for the meeting.

You must slaughter Keith in the Abolitionist.

And that £200,000! Talk of gangsters! Al Capone would have blushed.

G. Bernard Shaw

From Bernard Shaw.   4, WHITEHALL COURT (130) LONDON, S.W.1
                     PHONE: VICTORIA 3160.
                     TELEGRAMS: SOCIALIST. PARL-LONDO

20th February 1930.

My dear Hadwen,

    I cannot possibly engage myself for the 12th June. Heaven knows where I shall be then! Ever since H.G.Wells gave Pavlov, the Russian specialist on reflexes, a testimonial for humanity and for being adored by his dogs I have been tempted to take the platform again and give the public my own view of his book; but I should have to read it very carefully through before doing so; and that would take some time. I have only dipped into it so far; and the impression it left on me was that Pavlov would have seemed in the Ages of Faith to be a lunatic possessed by Satan, but that he had not brains enough to appreciate the cruelty and folly of what he spent 25 years in doing. If this impression has any validity it is time somebody made the world aware of it; for he is becoming almost as great an idol as Pasteur.

    I am very full of work this year, and likely to remain so until the Malvern Festival is over; so I amy not sanguine about being able to speak; but anyhow, if I can manage it, I have a theme ready.

                       Faithfully
                       G. Bernard Shaw

Dr Walter Hadwen,
Gloucester.

GBS lived at this address, Shaw's Corner, from 1906 to death in 1950.

Obviously GBS respected Hadwen and held him in high esteem. GBS is quoted as assessing Hadwen's comprehensive knowledge of a subject and his oratory as 'The Unanswerable Hadwen'

The other famous person to make Hadwen's acquaintance in 1911 was the visitation arranged for General Booth, founder of the Salvation Army, to meet Hadwen at his house. One assumes that they shared at least their common commitment to being teetotal and vegetarian. We do not know what other convictions they shared besides their Christian Faith nor the purpose of this visit a year before Booth died. There must have been much mutual admiration. Later, a newspaper report stated that the son of General Booth was summoned to the Worship Street Police Court, for not having his infant daughter vaccinated. He did not appear in court but wrote to say he had conscientious objections to the practice and the court decided on the mitigated penalty of five shillings. This may reflect his father's attitude to vaccination.

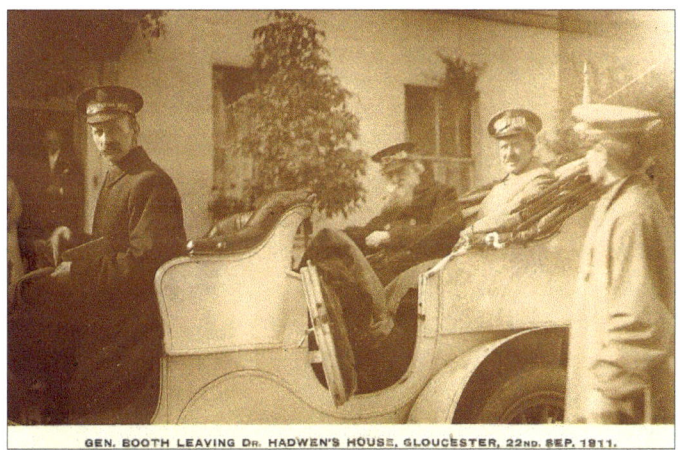

GEN. BOOTH LEAVING DR. HADWEN'S HOUSE, GLOUCESTER, 22ND. SEP. 1911.

Some time later, when Hadwen was invited by the secretary of Charing Cross Medical Society to give a lecture and then a debate on the subject of Experiments on Living Animals, a storm broke out as a result of a petition by the vivisection party. The original Hon Sec. who had organised the lecture had been suddenly replaced and the newly appointed Secretary informed Hadwen that the lecture had been cancelled. So much for freedom of speech! Hadwen stated that 'public speaking, however, forms my chief recreation from a busy practice'. It seems his enthusiasm and commitment to his cause was undaunted.

6
PERSONAL AND PROFESSIONAL MATTERS

Hadwen's letters to his mother gave detail of his activities, meetings, temperance lectures and two ambulance classes. One of these classes was to the men of the Great Western Railway, Gloucester, and had to take place on a Sunday afternoon, the only time the men were free. His classes were illustrated by reconstructed accidents. The women had a separate class. All this was done in his 'free time' and at no charge.

A holiday in 1903 presented Hadwen with the next challenge in the form of a cycling week with his daughter. They apparently covered over 500 miles and wishing to get back to Gloucester for the Sunday meeting, he and daughter cycled through the night. After 30 miles of pouring rain the daughter gave in and took a train back to Gloucester. Wet through Hadwen cycled on, a total of 120 miles, arriving also wet through. He had his usual cold bath by 9. 30. am, then breakfast and off to Albion Hall. The habit of a cold bath or shower was also recommended and practised by John Wesley; perhaps Hadwen felt this was good 'advice', it must have been at least invigorating. This episode illustrates that inertia was not Hadwen's forte, a holiday break was a physical challenge as well as giving pleasure.

That year Hadwen's father died at his house in Burnham. Within a few months his mother was knocked down by a brewer's dray, an unfortunate scenario for a teetotaller. She was unconscious for days and then made a limited recovery which allowed Hadwen to bring her back to his home in Gloucester and care for her. She had a poor quality of life for six more years and died age 96 years.

I have previously mentioned that, throughout his public and professional life, attempts were made to challenge Hadwen's views. In November 1908 a Nottingham doctor placed an anonymous letter in the *Nottingham Daily Express*. He was an opponent and made out that

Hadwen was a paid agitator. Eventually a reply was published to state Dr Hadwen had never accepted any fee for his addresses on the anti-vivisection cause. Again, an opponent in the USA claimed Hadwen's business was propaganda on which his livelihood depended. He made enemies by being critical of people who claimed falsehoods and in particular unproven cures for cancer.

In 1904 a charge was raised that Hadwen had certified a child's cause of death as being 'Disease of the Brain'. A local doctor started the rumour that the child really died of smallpox and Hadwen had attempted to conceal the fact that an unvaccinated child had died of smallpox. A letter denouncing Hadwen's action was brought to the attention of the city council, Hadwen felt he had to defend his name and professional reputation. Reading between the lines, this accusation caused great distress, particularly as Hadwen had no idea at the time that the child was unvaccinated. He became ill and a trial in Birmingham had to be postponed for a while. The hearing took place before Judge and Jury which resulted in his name and reputation being cleared, but he was only awarded a derisory farthing in damages, hardly an adequate redress. Each side was ordered to pay their own costs. The latter amounted to 100 guineas for Hadwen. The general feeling was that the damages awarded were so menial that the judgement reflected bias to the anti-vaccination movement. As a result of this case, Hadwen was invited by the Anti-Vaccination League to attend a meeting in London at the Westminster Palace Hotel in July 1904, where the officers and supporters of the League presented him with £160 to cover the legal costs involved. The Earl of Tankerville was in the chair for this occasion. The Earl shared the debating platform with Hadwen many times over the years and they became fond friends.

The year 1906 saw the appointment of the Royal Commission on Vivisection but Hadwen declined to appear and the BUAV was not represented. He felt that the members of the Commission would be prejudiced and evidence unfairly interpreted.

In November 1909 a 'so called' advertisement was placed in the *Citizen* newspaper ' Dr Hadwen desires to inform those parents who are anxious to make a declaration of conscientious objection to vaccination that he will be prepared to witness such declaration at his office, 139 Barton Street, on any day, except Thursday and Sunday from 9. 30 to 10 in the morning and 6 to 7 in the evening. All such declarations must be made before the child is four months old'.

No. 1a.

To PARENTS and GUARDIANS
How to Avoid Vaccination

THE VACCINATION ACT, 1907.

A form of declaration of conscientious objection must be obtained, either from the Vaccination Officer or from some other source, which must be **FILLED IN, IN INK,** except the date and signature. If the Vaccination Officer is also the Registrar of Births the exemption form could be applied for when the birth is registered. The address of the Vaccination Officer will be found on the vaccination paper given at registration of the birth of the child.

Then the **FATHER,** not the mother, must **TAKE THE FORM** to a Commissioner for Oaths, or a Justice of the Peace, or a Stipendiary Magistrate, and **MAKE A DECLARATION** of conscientious objection before him in the terms of the Form. This Declaration **must be made within four months of the birth of the child.** It is **useless** if made **later.**

The fee for the Declaration is generally 1/- at the Court and 2/- to a Commissioner.

WHEN THE DECLARATION HAS BEEN SIGNED by the Magistrate or Commissioner, **TAKE** or **SEND IT IMMEDIATELY,** by post or otherwise, **TO YOUR VACCINATION OFFICER.** It will be **OF NO USE** unless he gets it **WITHIN SEVEN DAYS** after its signature by the Commissioner or Magistrate. It is not necessary that application should be made at a Police Court; most Solicitors are Commissioners for Oaths, and will take your declaration without questioning you. **Some Magistrates will sign the declaration privately, when no fee can be charged.** No Magistrate has a right to question an applicant.

Forms of Declaration will be supplied free of charge by Dr. WALTER R. HADWEN, J.P., 139 Barton Street, Gloucester, who will be happy to sign them any day, except Sundays and Thursday Evenings, between the hours of 9 to 10 in the morning and 6 to 7 in the evening.

This type of advice was issued as a separate sheet but similar wording was used in the Citizen Newspaper and Dr Hadwen was accused of advertising

A letter from the Central Ethical Committee of the BMA stated that they had been asked to consider what was alleged to be an advertisement, appearing in a local newspaper. (see the copy of the offending leaflet).

Hadwen replied to the effect that this pettiness characterises some members of the profession and he was not surprised at the sinister construction placed upon his announcement which, in Hadwen's view, enabled 'conscious' objectors (especially the working classes) to know when and where they can get their declarations witnessed free of charge etc. This was another irksome challenge by the local profession which must have caused more hurt. However, on investigation and full correspondence on the matter, the outcome was that the announcement did not technically breach medical ethics.

Hadwen courted controversy again in 1909 when the cause of Malta Fever (Brucellosis) was found to be prevented by stopping consumption of goat's milk on the island. Once more he produced figures to show that a fall in incidence of 50% was due to improved sanitation not the prohibition of goat's milk. He closely looked into what facts could be ascertained at the time and came out against the evidence by Colonel Bruce that the disease was due to a micrococcus found in unpasteurised goat's milk. He had travelled to Malta to investigate the problem.

Hadwen strengthened his philosophy by an intense study of the Registrar-General's annual statistics. He made his analyses on 5-yearly figures. Mainly he argued that figures showed that zymotic disease decreased in prevalence with improved sanitation, as proposed by the Public Health Act 1875 and would see the nation's health improve without resort to vaccination measures. Hadwen produced a pamphlet with all the statistics to illustrate his argument and circulated it to every doctor in 'the kingdom'. There followed prolonged correspondence again within the *BMJ* as they interpreted the statistics to suit their view. In the event, Sir David Bruce's work on the micrococcus as a cause of Malta Fever was officially recognised.

In 1913 Hadwen was invited to give evidence before the legislative council of the Isle of Man on the subject of granting the inhabitants conscientious objection to vaccination. The debate was whether to allow this human right as was now the case on the mainland. He gave lengthy evidence and was closely questioned but he was the only anti-vaccinationist called to give evidence. Three other members of the medical profession made the case for compulsory vaccination. Despite this, the outcome was that the 'Conscience Clause' was adopted by the Isle of Man legislature. More correspondence ensued and was published about the way Hadwen's evidence was reported.

7
COMMUNICATION AND CORRESPONDENCE

IF, FOR NOTHING ELSE, Hadwen should be remembered for the amazing output of the written word both to relatives, friends and also manuscripts supporting his campaigns. Amongst all he wrote there are very few examples of his handwriting apart from signatures on flyleaves of presentation books, etc

The authors of *Hadwen of Gloucester* include copy of letters between Hadwen and his family, especially when he was training in London. There are also 'poems' and I have already mentioned the poem of nineteen verses attacking his local MP.

Apparently he never had secretarial assistance specifically in his Gloucester practice. All his correspondence would have been hand written. He had a talent for sketching which he used on some personal Christmas greeting cards. I was told that one of the senior partners had a collection of Hadwen's anatomical sketches from his anatomy studies at medical school but somehow these have been misplaced and unlikely to resurface.

I have included the marvellous examples of his artistic skill. The envelopes are addressed to John, his brother, and they show his talent. John was born in 1857, it is said he kept a school for the sons of Officers in the Army and Navy at Wandsworth Common. Later he went to Philadelphia and became Secretary of the London Association for the Protection of Trade. He married Sarah Coote in 1881. I have tried a search of passenger lists on 'Ancestry' website to see if it is possible to be more accurate over his travels but no trace was found. His date of death is not accurately recorded but apparently he died back in UK. These sketches seem to be mainly dated 1876 when John was at Bedford House School. It may be he was teaching there, but it is said Hadwen wrote to his brother on some family matters at that time from Reading. I have a scrap book which I

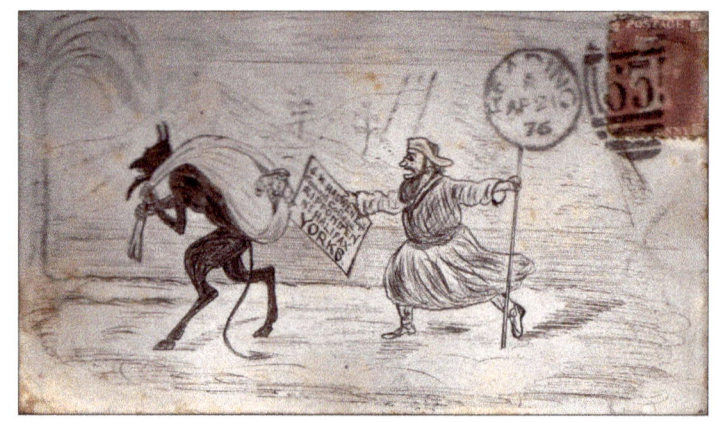
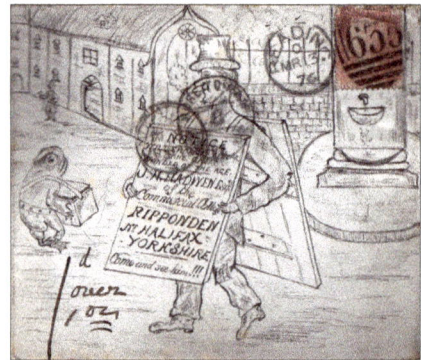
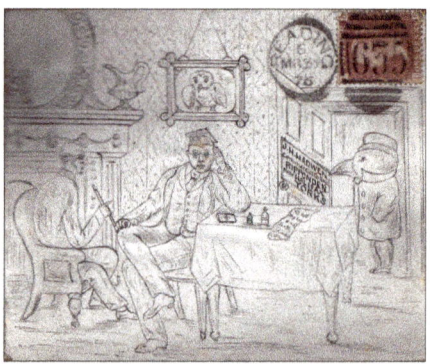
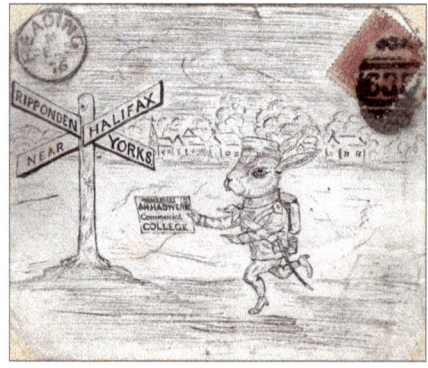
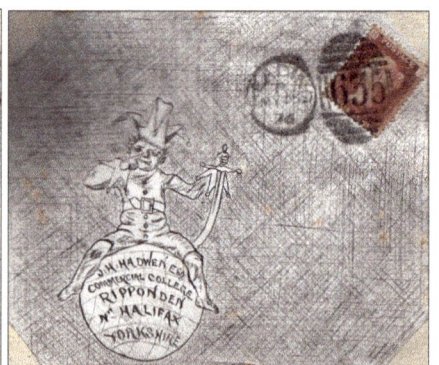
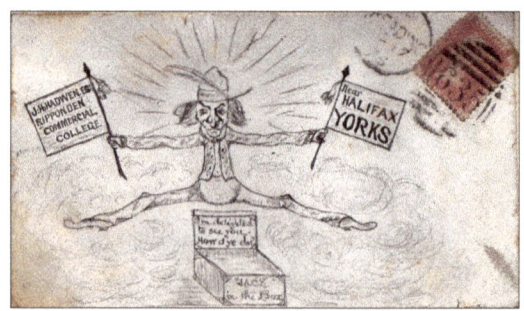

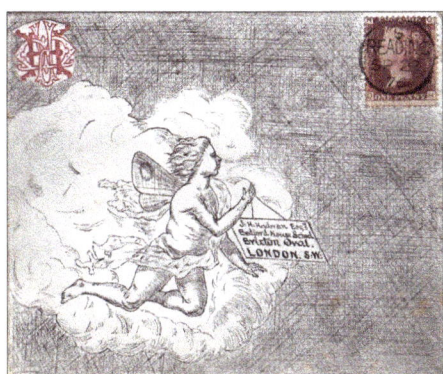

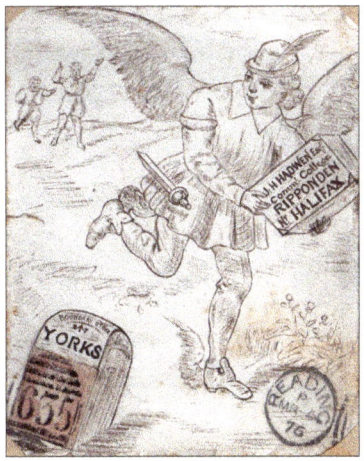

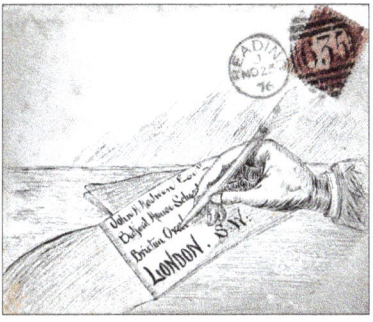

The final envelope shows that realistic drawings of animals was part of Hadwen's talent and this is of his pet dog 'Fan', presumably named from the dog tail's wag!! Also a mini-photo of John found in the back of the Album.

> You wish a bright New Year?
> Then — You must make it.
> It offers you a tear?
> Then — bravely take it.
> Try to shed some beams of light
> Among those whose day is night,
> And the year will then be bright,
> But — You must make it.
>
> There is work enough to do.
> But — You must do it;
> Success is certain too
> But — You must woo it.
> If you lack the needed skill,
> It is useless sitting still,
> You can train the force of will,
> If — You will do it.
>
> Walter R Hadwen

An example of Hadwen's handwriting and New Year greeting

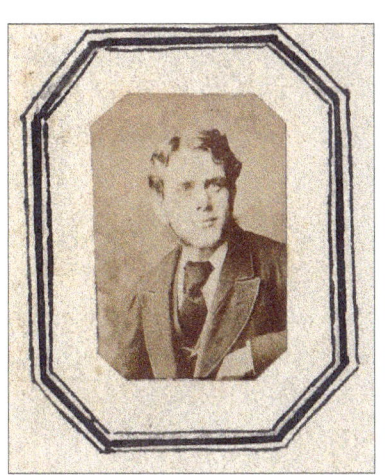

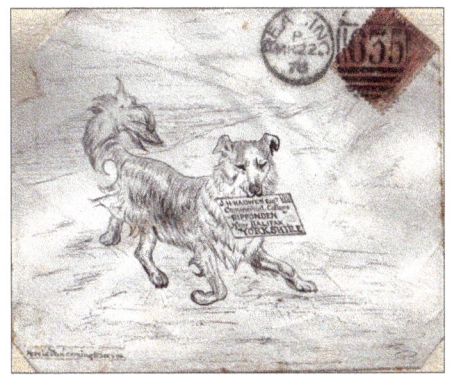

believe was John's with the insignia of the school displayed. It seems he also attended the Commercial College, Ripponden, near Halifax. So these are all originals scanned on to these pages.

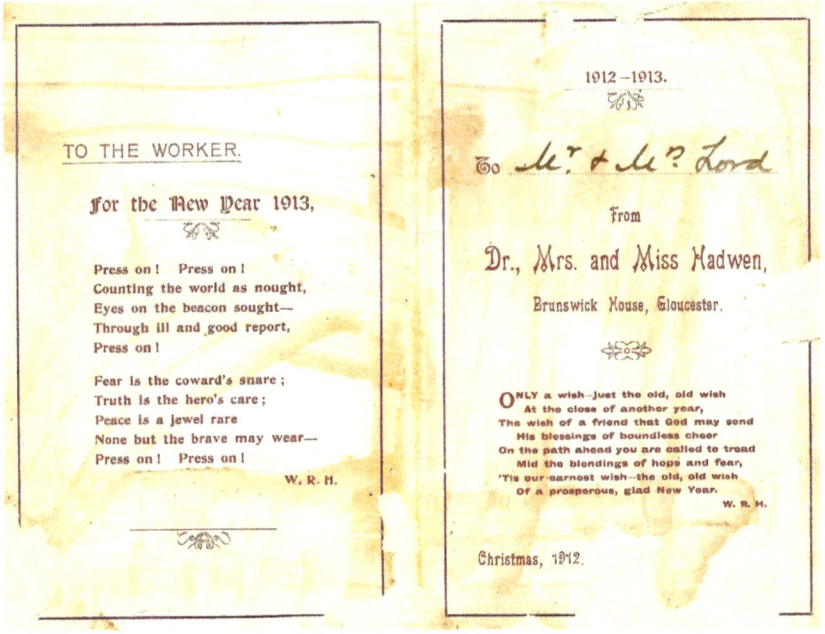

1912 Greeting Card for the New Year all verses composed by Hadwen

October 13th 1905.

Dear Mr Hall,

I only heard yesterday of the fact that your dear wife had fallen asleep through Jesus. I was greatly surprised and was very grieved for you. But for the poor sufferer it is indeed a happy release. She is with the Lord now - with the one she loved so well, and who loved her. May God, in his grace grant that you may be strengthened by this trial which all of you must feel keenly. We cannot always understand the why and wherefores of these things, but we may rest assured that He does all things well, and that everything is according to His own love and purpose. The day will come when we shall understand it all when we see His face and know even as we are known.

With true, deep sympathy in your affliction and sorrow.

Believe me

Very truly Yours,

Walter R Hadwen.

A rare example of a letter of a handwritten letter by Hadwen expressing sympathy to a friend (transcript on page opposite)

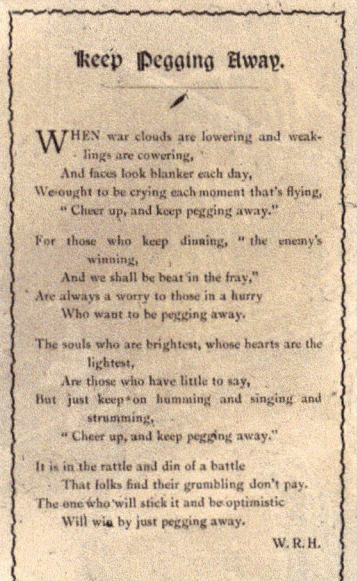

Other examples of Hadwen composing a Hymn and an encouraging poem to anyone to overcome any difficulty.

In attempting to give some idea of Hadwen's output both by word of mouth and in his writing I have listed in 'Bibliography' the books he wrote entirely himself as well as the *Premature Burial* which he edited. I have summarised these volumes and given detail for reference. The listing also gives the places where lectures were given to indicate how much he travelled to speak in public in the UK, never mind extra lectures and notes whilst abroad. I have tried, in another chapter, to document Hadwen's travels, which included two visits to America. He sent articles of his adventures back to the local *Citizen* newspaper recording events in some detail.

For some years I have had in my possession two examples of Hadwen's recorded voice. They are ten half inch shellac 78rpm recordings under the label 'Standard' British Made. I believe this to be a private recording which would be quite innovative in the first half of the 20th century. It is undated but the subject is 'The Case against Vivisection From the Moral Standpoint'. The reverse side is 'From the Medical Standpoint'. The recording is by 'Dr W. R. Hadwen, J. P. ' I have been able to get the voice recording enhanced by a BBC technician and now transcribed. We have no information as to where a recording studio, as such, was and whether this project was financed by the BUAV.

I can only comment on the wisdom of the 'Moral Standpoint' in that the first two paragraphs are prophetic when considering Hitler's morals in the Second World War

THE CASE AGAINST VIVISECTION. FROM THE MORAL STANDPOINT.
(Transcribed from the recording)

There are two main points to be considered in coming to a conclusion upon the moral aspects of the vivisection question.

First, is there strong justification for taking advantage of the weak? If this be admitted, we will be justified in vivisecting a human baby, in taking advantage of the poor in hospitals or in experimenting upon the inmates of our asylums.

Second, are we justified in doing evil so that good may come. If so, there is no wickedness under the sun for which an excuse could not be found. It would justify the thumbscrew and the rack and every normative practice in the middle ages to wrest secrets from human prisoners.

It is urged that, in as much as animals have to be slaughtered for food, vivisection is justifiable in the interests of humanity. Not so, when a butcher seeks to slay his victim as expeditiously as possible, whereas a vivisector keeps his victim alive as long as he can, until the result of the experiment is known.

Animals have rights. This is now recognised by law, and unquestionably the least of all rights is to be spared the worst of all wrongs.

Is vivisection the worst of all wrongs? Suggest that similar experiments be performed on human beings that are performed on animals, and everyone will shrink in horror from the proposition. It is recognised as something worse than death.

The Physiologist tampers with the natural functions of an animal's body to gain knowledge of little or no value to the human subject. He cuts out organs or parts of organs, ties ducts controlling vital processes, destroys portions of the brain, inserts gallstones in the gall bladder, deposits artificial tumours in the brain, paints or varnishes the animal body, injects the products of disease into the bloodstream, feeds the animal with loathsome and unnatural substances, or omits from its diet some element which he knows to be essential to its existence, then watches day by day the results of these proceedings.

The assertion that vivisection does not involve much suffering in England is merely a tribute to the strength of our anti-vivisection agitation. It conceals an obvious fact, namely that the British law allows cruelty and protects the vivisector. The root principle of our struggle on behalf of speechless and defenceless animals lies in the fact that the practice is immoral, and we demand its abolition. It ought not to be linked up with a civilised and prophetically Christian State.

Pray enrol yourself as a member of the British Union, 32 Charing Cross, London, South West One. There are branches all over Great Britain, Ireland and in the Colonies; it being the largest Anti-Vivisection Society in the World.

THE CASE AGAINST VIVISECTION. FROM THE MEDICAL STANDPOINT.

(Again transcribed from the recording)

Vivisection is not only cruel, it is utterly useless. Medical students are taught that practically all the knowledge upon which the practice of medicine and surgery stands, has come through a pathway of experimentation upon living animals. The knowledge of the circulation of the blood is claimed as one of its triumphs, but when Harvey, at the close of his career, was asked by his biographer, the Hon. Robert Boyle, what really led him to believe that the blood circulated, he replied that it was his examination of the valves in the veins of a dead subject.

Sir Charles Bell, who discovered the double action of the spinal nerves, wrote decisively that experiments have never been the means of discovery. Even Claude Bernard, the famous vivisector, wrote at the end of his life of the vivisectors' empty hands and mouths full of promises. That has indeed always been the condition of the vivisector. It was a discussion between two eminent surgeons upon the brain's centres revealing a great discrepancy between the conclusions of different vivisectors concerning the same experiments, that first showed me the utter fallacy of this method of investigation.

The modern, insane fashion of inoculating disease poisons into the system not only to fight disease but under the idea that of protecting against diseases we may never encounter, owes its origin and progress entirely to vivisection. The method is unnatural and unscientific for its results cannot be gauged nor are they based upon trustworthy statistical data. The system of inoculation is supported by tremendous commercial interests which lie at the back of it, but the terrible results on human health and life are concealed until they become so glaring that the truth leaks out as in the deaths from encephalitis consequent on vaccination.

Experimentation on living animals is gravely misleading owing to the fact that you cannot reason from an animal to a man, the differences both anatomically and physiologically being so great. To claim the progress of surgery owes its advances to vivisection is a pure myth.

Lawson Tait, perhaps one of the greatest and most original surgeons who ever lived, declared 'vivisection had done nothing for surgery but lead to horrible bungling'. Some day medical men will wipe out this foul blot on the page of their proud history and will return to the sound principles propounded by Hippocrates some 500 years BC.

A long, exhaustive study of this subject has convinced me that nothing whatever has been achieved by vivisection either in the amelioration or cure of any human disease.

It is urged that, in as much as animals have to be slaughtered for food, vivisection is justifiable in the interests of humanity. Not so, when a butcher seeks to slay his victim as expeditiously as possible, whereas a vivisector keeps his victim alive as long as he can, until the result of the experiment is known.

Is vivisection the worst of all wrongs? Suggest that similar experiments be performed on human beings that are performed on animals, and everyone will shrink in horror from the proposition. It is recognised as something worse than death.

The physiologist tampers with the natural functions of an animal's body to gain knowledge of little or no value to the human subject. He cuts out organs or parts of organs, ties ducts controlling vital processes, destroys portions of the brain, inserts gallstones in the gall bladder, deposits artificial tumours in the brain, paints or varnishes the animal's body, injects the products of disease into the bloodstream, feeds the animal with loathsome and unnatural substances, or omits from its diet some element which he knows to be essential to its existence, then watches day by day the results of these proceedings.

The assertion that vivisection does not involve much suffering in England is merely a tribute to the strength of our anti vivisection agitation. It conceals an obvious fact, namely that the British Law allows cruelty and protects the vivisector. The root principle of our struggle on behalf of speechless and defenceless animals lies in the fact that the practice is immoral, and we demand its abolition. It ought not to be linked up with a civilised and prophetically Christian State.

Pray enrol yourself as a member of the British Union, 32 Charing Cross, London South West One. There are branches all over Great Britain, Ireland and in the Colonies; it being the largest Anti-Vivisection Society in the World.

The Partners and the Medical Practice that inherited Hadwen's patients must be unique in having the actual recorded voice of Hadwen, the founder, making his appeal to the public.

To have these recordings and hear the voice you can capture the effect he would have on an audience or individual. A reporter for the *Citizen* newspaper gave this opinion in 1896 of Hadwen's anti-vaccination talk at the Old Corn Exchange which stood on the Cross in Gloucester opposite the Bell Hotel

'What a spate of oratory it was, to be sure! There came a point in the oration when every alternate period seemed to be working up to a peroration; but on and on the doctor went, waxing warmer and warmer and almost literally spitting out his loathing and contempt for the practitioners of the Jennerian Cult. It was a terrific *tour de force*, delivered in the prime of his strength and intellectual vigour, as may well be imagined by those who, in later years, have been enthralled for a couple of hours without a break as the doctor painted his vivid prose pictures of his travels in many lands'.

When performing a search in the *British Medical Journal* website, I found that there were no fewer than 276 references mentioning Hadwen. Many were letters, responses and debate over controversial medical topics but this number gives some idea of Hadwen's commitment to his causes and defence of his views. Many copies of public talks and lectures are open for inspection online from the Wellcome Trust Library.

8
JOHN HADWEN, KNOWN AS 'JACK'
BORN 1883

THERE IS NO DETAIL of John's early life and education but we have some information of his attending the local Crypt Grammar School in Gloucester. The school record shows that he entered at the age of thirteen years in the first term of 1897 and left in the first term of 1901. He went on to St. Bartholomew's Medical School, London University. His qualifications were M. B. , B. S. , B. Sc. Detail is not clear but it would appear he obtained a position as a ship's doctor aboard the P&O Line, the S. S. Arabia. Archive letters confirm his travels to China and Japan (Kyoto) and India. A Japanese acquaintance writes to ask Jack to continue contact as he was studying English, dated August 1908. Several unused postcards handed to me along with this letter from Japan seem to indicate Jack visited Marseille, Bombay and Nanking (showing stone horse sculptures on the approach to the Xiao Ling Mausoleum). A letter to Una (his sister) from Marseille tells of having to look after the crew and three doctors from P&O ships all ill with fever. He had an extra trip aboard the *Oriental* to assist with delivery of mail to Aden. He had obviously been able to take time out to tour Japan in some detail. He hints at this time, when he is due back in UK around 1908 that he was happy to help his father as a locum.

However, on returning home he took the competitive Royal Naval Medical Examination in 1909. Thirty-two candidates competed for fifteen positions and John came fifth in total marks and was accepted. He went for further training at the Royal Naval Hospital in Haslar, Gosport and this was followed by six months aboard 'HMS Dominion'. From there he joined *HMS Cornwallis* in the Mediterranean for fifteen months. He was repatriated to RNH Hasler for a further nine months.

The year 1914 saw the beginning of the war and active service when he was appointed to serve on *HMS King Edward VII*, described

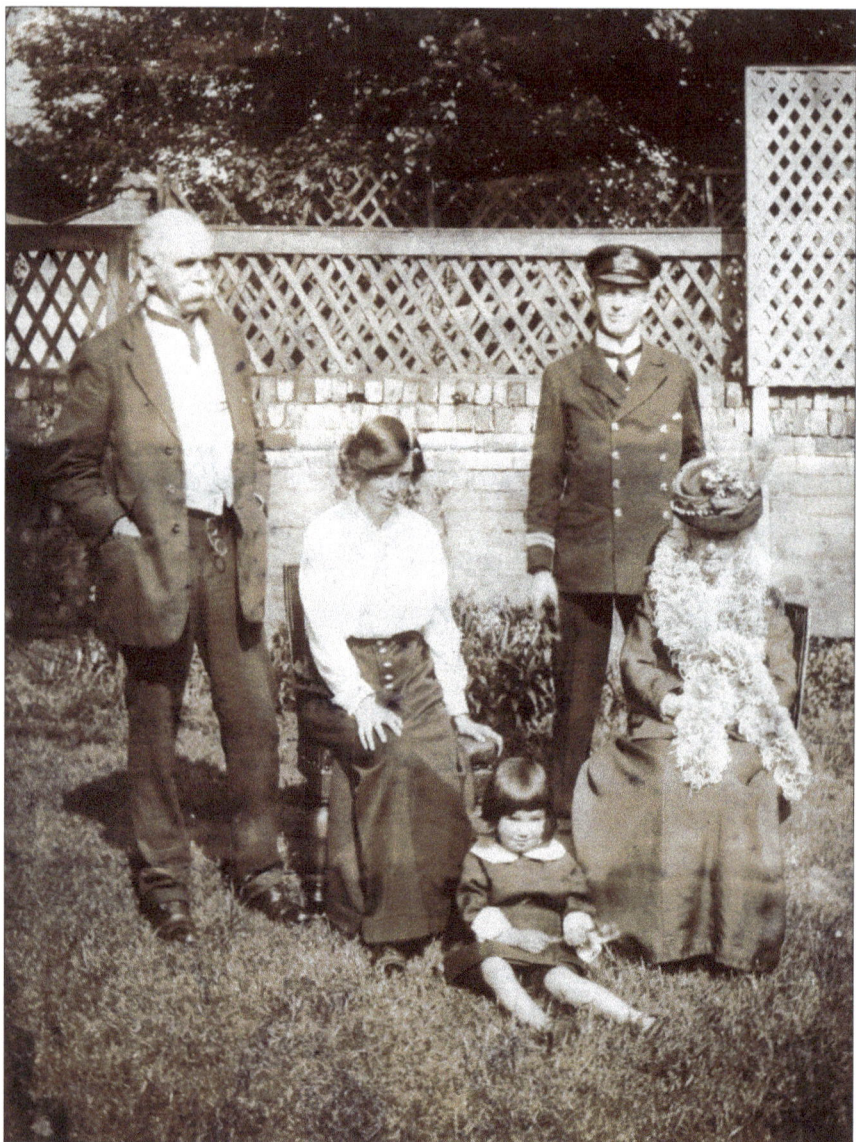

This photo is the only one I have found to show the Hadwen Family. L to R: Dr Walter Hadwen, Una (seated) with daughter Eulalie on grass, 'Jack' Hadwen in uniform and Mrs Alice Hadwen.

as a pre-dreadnaught battleship. Originally this vessel was the flagship of the 'Atlantic Fleet' but after reorganisations this became designated as 'Grand Fleet'. It is reported that to meet his ship Jack had to travel on *HMS Africa*, another battleship, but the two ships failed to meet! Admiralty records make no mention of him having to stay on *HMS*

Africa and the official record states he served on *HMS King Edward VII* for at least six months. Discrepancies in data hint that either he stayed on the *Africa* or transferred to *HMS Caesar*. From November 1915 he served on *HMS Aphis* only launched in September of that year. This was one of four gunboats based in Port Said where he experienced the First Battle of Gaza. In undated correspondence he also mentions serving on the gunboat *HMS Ladybird*. Jack was then transferred to *HMS City of Oxford* in October 1917 and finally *HMS Lancaster* from 2 March 1918. This ship was classed as an armoured cruiser and was eventually assigned to the Pacific Fleet and became the flagship of the Eastern Squadron in 1918.

I have a handwritten letter from one of Jack's friends dated 6 December, 1918 from the Island of Taboga, Gulf of Panama. He had exchanged reading material with Jack and obviously had no idea of Jack's last voyage in the *Lancaster*. Another note to Mrs Hadwen from Jack in Cairo, but undated, is quite revealing. I surmise that the sister Gracie gives Jack concern over her very restricted self-imposed vegetarian diet. He makes reference to a story in a copy of the *Abolitionist* about the Argumentative Club being very pleasantly written, and reference to a charming young naval officer in that article. The author was Hadwen Snr. and this inclusion of the naval officer is more fully explored in Hadwen's book, *The Difficulties of Dr Deguerre*, a summary of which I have included in Appendices at the end of the book. Jack hints that he would be safer from action if he was back in the North Sea or Mesopotamia. He states he is fit and well and life agreeable, then finishes with, 'I send my love and remain your affectionate son'. A letter to sister Una, again undated, acknowledges the new arrival of her selected reading material and he, in return, had sent her a sample of Egyptian embroidery. He claims to have two certified genuine scarabs removed from Egyptian tombs dated about 1500BC. Another requests from Una specific books he requires and mention is made of receiving a box with pipe and cigarettes from Princess Mary (sometimes these appear still complete in Antique fairs). A longer letter to Hadwen Snr. in response to one Jack had received from his father with a couple of copies of the *Abolitionist*. Jack feels able to express a view that 'Darwin's theory of evolution by natural selection' forms a useful hypothesis and a good explanation of the facts of the organic world'. Jack also relates that he has met one or two old contacts, one of whom had been decorated with a Military Cross. He reflects on how men who have never left their villages or factories react to living

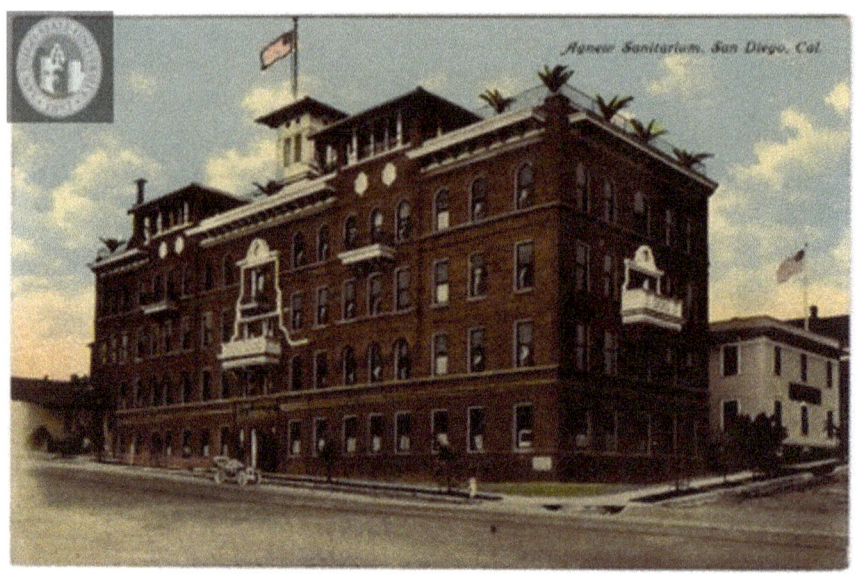

The Agnew Sanitarium in San Diego to where Jack was transferred from HMS Lancaster, and where he died

in the open and enforced cleanliness and sobriety, and admires their cheerfulness and readiness to serve. He states that the amount of sickness is negligible. It is not surprising that in wartime letters were undated as part of censorship. Whilst in Cairo, there was no mention of an epidemic.

By 1918 it seems that Jack was the chief in Medical Command of three vessels which included the *HMS Lancaster*. He was confronted by a severe outbreak of influenza (the pandemic which became known as 'Spanish Flu')

In London, Hadwen Snr. was to attend a meeting to discuss the subject of animal experiments, travelling from Gloucester at 7. 15am and arriving Paddington 10. 30am. Met by his secretary, he ordered a taxi to get to the Admiralty, the BUAV HQ being directly opposite. He informed Miss Kidd that he had had a cable from San Diego stating that Jack was dangerously ill. He added 'They usually break things gradually. It probably means that he is dead. I must call and enquire.' He shortly returned to BUAV offices and broke down, repeating 'my only son!' He sent a telegram back to his wife and the family all heard the news. Grief was exacerbated by the family receiving letters from Jack posted from various ports before his illness and death, some stating he looked forward to a home-coming. These events are described in detail in the book by Kidd but a specific date has been omitted of this tragic day. I have a copy of a letter of notification from the Admiralty to Hadwen Snr. in Gloucester dated 24 October 1918. This letter states that 'The Lords Commissioners of the Admiralty have commanded that you be informed that a telegram had been received stating that your son, Surgeon-Lieutenant-Commander John Hadwen died in St. Agnew Hospital, Santiago' on 23rd October 1918, further information was to follow. The error in this letter stating 'Santiago' rather than 'San Diego' California can possibly be accounted for by the number of 'casualties' to be notified at this late stage of the war. Once more accuracy of date of death is excluded in Kidd's book.

There follow several letters to pay tribute to Jack. Some already are in print in Hadwen's biography. The first on 25 October, 1918 from P. H. Colomb, Rear-Admiral, *HMS Lancaster*, which states that Jack had treated and brought back to health and safety some 200 to 300 patients. Officers and men recognised his service and sacrifice. Jack was charming and popular. His funeral was attended by every officer that could get away and every man that could be spared. Also attending were members of the crew and Admiral Fullam of an American battleship *Oregon* in port at the time. The original letter is in my archive. A tribute is sent from the Chaplain on 28 October. Again, I have the original, handwritten and on plain personal stationery giving more detail. The ship was on its way to Canada for a refit, a remark indicates that influenza had reached the West Coast of America, the infection may have been picked up in Calleo (Peru's chief seaport) or Payta (sometimes spelt Paita also in Peru). The sick list rose to 200 and the burden of care fell on Jack's shoulders as his junior doctor had already fallen ill. Jack delayed reporting ill with a temperature of 103 degrees, he contracted pneumonia. Soon he was moved from his own cabin to the Captain's bridge cabin to make him more comfortable.

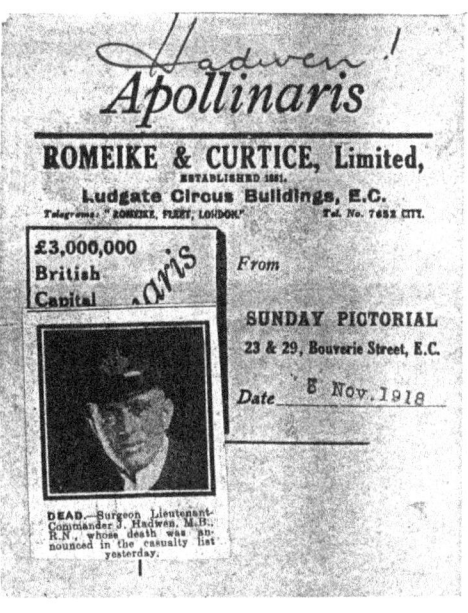

One of several identical announcements of Jack's death

Although he recognised his medical symptoms he was optimistic about convalescence in California, the next port of call being San Diego. On landing there, he was immediately transferred to St. Agnew Hospital where he received every care and attention from the USA Naval Medical Staff and specialist nurses. He started to improve but shortly became semi-conscious. The sailing of HMS *Lancaster* was postponed until the outcome of his condition was known. Oxygen had been administered but despite a short 'rally' he died at 11. 45 am. (Dates in this letter do not tally with official records and are confusing). Jack's body was laid to rest in the beautiful Greenwood cemetery overlooking the harbour, with full naval honours, and touching remarks were made by local inhabitants. The Chaplain states that Jack loved his country and that he was faithful to his duty even unto death. Everyone spoke admiringly of him.

Recently I have obtained up to date images of the gravestone and its position in the cemetery with a variety of trees including tall palms.

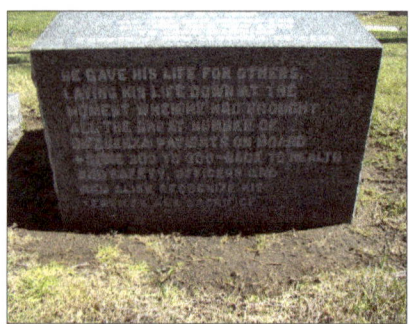 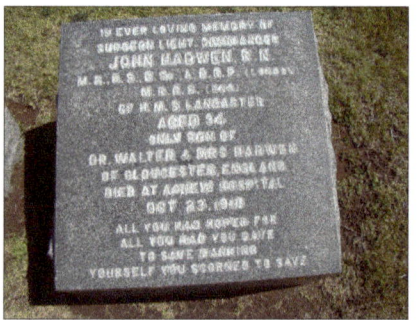

Inscription reads 'He gave his life for others, laying his life down at the moment when he had brought all the great number of influenza patients on board-some 200-300-back to health and safety, officers and men alike recognise his services and sacrifice. Rear Admiral P.H.Colomb. R.N.
'All you had hoped for, All you had you gave to save mankind, yourself you scorned to save'.

This tragic event, taking place so far from Jack's home country was made even worse when subsequent actions came to Dr Hadwen's notice. A handwritten letter from Jack's close colleague, the staff paymaster, states that the Flag Captain was to request a posthumous recognition from the Admiralty to mark Jack's selfless devotion to his patients. However this never came to pass. It was stated that his private gear and books were transferred with him to the hospital. The last tribute describes Jack as vivacious, cheerful and full of mirth and of a rare intelligence.

Then, to quote 'His uniform and plain clothes are, by service custom, being sold on the ship. This included his cap, sword and belt, for the funeral they were laid on the coffin. I ask that I keep a plain pewter napkin ring of his as a memento.'

The Captain of HMS Lancaster in a letter to Dr Hadwen stated 'He was very popular with both officers and men and I can assure you that we feel his loss very greatly and sympathise with his family very genuinely.'

Subsequently the Staff paymaster informed Dr. Hadwen that the 'gear' was all sold and produced the sum of £75.

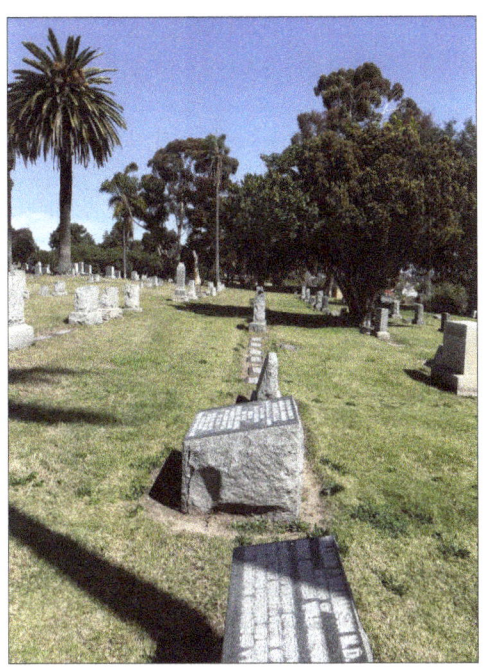

Greenwood Memorial Park, San Diego

In November an official letter from the Admiralty confirmed that Jack's 'effects' had been sold except for articles of personal value and a gun and sporting gear. Dr. Hadwen was asked to intimate his wishes as to the disposal of the latter.

The response from Hadwen was in anger and distress at events. A handwritten reply of November 8th shows his grief.

> I am at a loss to understand by what authority the effects of my son have been sold without my authority and sanction. What is included under that term and what distinction is drawn between his effects and articles of personal value? Do I understand that his boxes have been ransacked and their contents disposed of at the direction of somebody on board HMS Lancaster?

This letter is followed by the Admiralty statement that :-

Regulations allow the Commanding Officer of a ship full discretionary power to dispose of the deceased effects as he may think best, subject only to the reservation that the private books and papers are to be sealed up for transmission to the legal representative. In the exercise of that discretion, the distance of the vessel from the deceased family is taken into account and it is to be assumed that this circumstance and the difficulties of transport weighed with the Commanding Officer in determining his action in this particular case.

A further letter to the Admiralty states

I can neither do nor say anything until I know what articles have been sold. I have no objection to the 'gun and sporting gear' being disposed of as I have no use for them. If not sold they can be forwarded to me with the other effects. My son's boxes contained the accumulation and collection of four years; owing to difficulties of transit he was not able to get them home during the period of the war, and before leaving on his last voyage, he gave verbal instructions as to disposal of their contents, in case anything happened to him. I am therefore considerably concerned about them.

We have no further evidence of response or otherwise to this dilemma, only an Admiralty Official report on the circumstance of Jack's death which adds nothing new.

There is a touching note from a resident in San Diego who had Navy connections, 'I will keep an eye on his grave for his mother's sake, if he has one, although, here, graves are not allowed to be absolutely neglected, when you buy your plot, part of the price is devoted to upkeep by the cemetery authorities'.

It is likely that the Admiralty paid for the burial plot and the erection of the gravestone. I have examples of cuttings announcing Jack's death from various newspapers including the *Bristol Times*, Gloucester Echo, *Sunday Pictorial, Daily Graphic, Birmingham Post.*

In *First Impressions of America* Hadwen does not speak of visiting his son's grave in San Diego when he made his tour in 1921, but we know that he availed himself of the opportunity and laid family wreaths by the grave which had been kept well tended. Hadwen thought it a handsome monument but had dreaded the visit and that, in the end, he would have to leave the grave behind. He learnt from friends in San Diego how large and impressive the funeral had been, and another doctor reported to him that '38 of the ships crew were very ill indeed and had Jack gone to bed as they had wanted him to do (and his assistant had done) these men would have gone under. He attended to them night and day, and stuck to his post until he was simply exhausted, and didn't stand a dog's chance'.

The so-called 'Spanish Flu' Pandemic has been the subject of research, and evidence seems to show that the avian virus mutated to produce catastrophic symptoms in humans. There was a secondary phase of influenza towards the end of 1918 which caused more pronounced symptoms with very high temperature, headache, cough shortly producing pus and blood in the sputum, pneumonia and cyanosis, vomiting, diarrhoea and sudden collapse, which completed the patient's demise. The spread of the disease was hastened by troop movements and in particular the confines and close contact between personnel in ships. The history of illness of troops aboard *USS Leviathan* was a prime example. Peculiarly the infection seemed to hit the younger and fitter age group rather than infants and elderly. Medical officers, nurses and hospital facilities were overwhelmed. Towards the end of the war in France, there were major problems of coping in the huge transit camp in Étaples. All this happened before viruses had been identified by using the electron microscope and no antibiotics had been discovered. Jack Hadwen had all the risk factors, age group, close contact with the infection with overcrowding, meaning isolation of cases under his care was impossible on board his ship. The timing of his infection means it is very likely that he and his men were exposed to the later more virulent second wave of influenza. It may be that the infection was brought on board by any crew member visiting a port on leave on the final journey.

In Kidd's biography no mention is made of evidence of a similar epidemic in Gloucester at that time nor of it restricting Walter Hadwen's activities.

9
THE GREAT 'SMALLPOX' SCARE
1923

REMEMBERING THAT the electron microscope was not developed fully until the late 1930s, arguments about infection and its causes were not completely resolved, even if suspected, until a particle smaller than a bacterium, a 'virus', could be identified. It took until 1929 for the League of Nations Health Organisation to agree that there should be a revised disease classification of two specific diseases, *Variola major* (Smallpox) and *Variola minor* (Mild Smallpox), known originally as Alastrim. It was only in 1948 that the specificity of *variola minor* v *major* was confirmed in the laboratory. Other descriptive names used for this less severe disease were, White Pox, Kaffir pox, Cuban itch, West Indian Pox, Milk Pox and pseudovariola.

There was confusion at all levels in the profession as to the accuracy of smallpox diagnosis or any variant. The Chief Medical Officer, Sir George Newman, felt that Alastrim was the same disease as smallpox, and a new effort was initiated to control any outbreak by vaccination. Of course this was not a popular move in Gloucester.

Previously, in 1901, a mild form of smallpox had been described elsewhere and it was noted that on transmission within a community there was no evidence that the infection altered to become the more familiar and deadly true smallpox. All this debate was important as Gloucester citizens were treated like lepers when travelling away from the city. Some tourists took to wearing improvised masks when going through the city (this may be apocryphal or originated as a scare story in the Press!).

Once more, the rumour was spread in the community, and not for the first time, that Hadwen had gone to a nearby town at night and secretly been vaccinated. Hadwen had to publicly refute such a report.

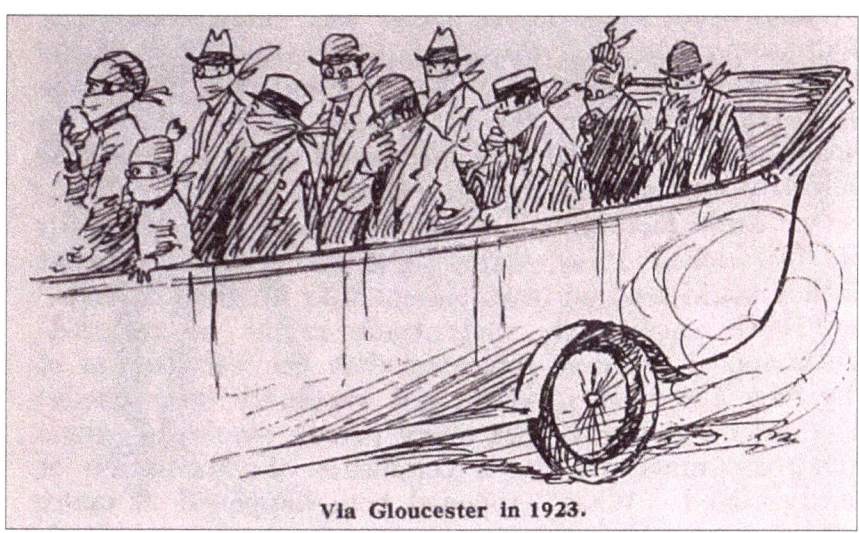
Via Gloucester in 1923.

Masks to prevent infection when travelling through Gloucester

In the Summer of 1923 Gloucester was said to be free of Smallpox. Shortly after this declaration, the Officials from the Ministry of Health checked records and found dozens of unreported smallpox cases in Gloucester and so further observation and care was taken to record suspicious smallpox cases.

This is where confusion started as to what defined the disease local doctors were diagnosing and notifying to the authorities. Similar outbreaks were being recorded in the Midlands.

There had been attempts to persuade the local population to be vaccinated, but because of the historic resistance to such a procedure fears were raised that many local people (both adults and children) were unvaccinated and therefore at risk. In the previous three years only 10% of babies in Gloucester had been vaccinated.

The authorities were quick to jump to conclusions and announced that this was another smallpox outbreak. To prevent spread of the disease isolation was the only answer. Memories of the 1896 smallpox outbreak surfaced and the worst scenario was envisaged. The old arguments and prejudices were ignited.

Hadwen was able to examine the 'patients' and their rash and, like some other medical practitioners, was sure this was not smallpox but chickenpox. This was a much milder disease but still with risks. The Ministry Medical Officers, with specialist knowledge of smallpox, were not to be deterred and were adamant that they were dealing with a new smallpox outbreak.

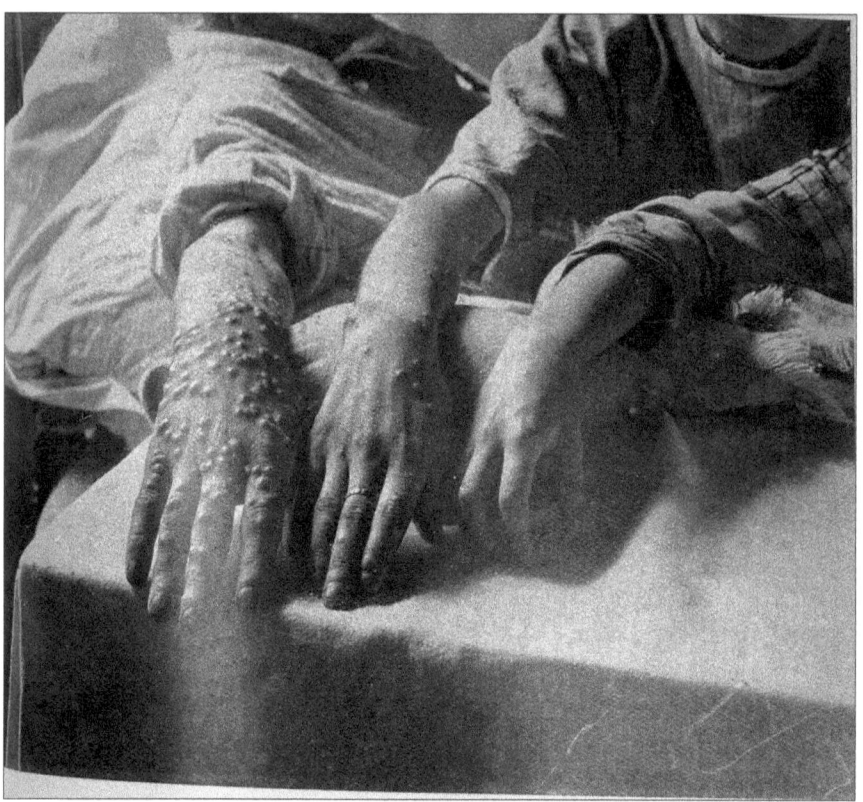

Comparative cases from L to R- Smallpox, Mild Smallpox and Chickenpox

Hadwen was again involved in controversy. Those who opposed him realised, once more, that they were up against a charismatic man whose views on smallpox had gained national prominence. It was said that Hadwen himself had notified a few cases he had seen as being genuine cases of smallpox. Later, because he then sided with some of his medical colleagues who agreed that most cases seen were really chickenpox, his old enemies were intent on ruining his reputation, as they thought him wrong and were convinced they were dealing with smallpox.

A report on 16 June 1923 stated that rumours of a smallpox outbreak were greatly exaggerated. There was hearsay that several hundred cases of smallpox were in the isolation hospitals, but Dr Bibby, the city Medical officer, confirmed to reporters that there were only sixteen cases of smallpox currently under treatment and four fresh cases just notified. They were being treated in the Gloucester Isolation Hospital at Over. He also stated that four nurses had been appointed and were waiting to attend referred cases to the Brockworth Aerodrome facility; whether this included the Matron and deputy Matron is not clear. Despite the conclusion by the local Public Health Officers that this was chickenpox, the advice from the Ministry was that preparations were to be made to isolate all those with symptoms in the old hangar belonging to the Gloucester Aircraft Company, Brockworth as a temporary 'overflow' facility.

These officials convened a meeting in the Guildhall with the local doctors on 13 June, 1923. 27 doctors were induced to sign a manifesto stating there were a large number of cases of smallpox existing in the city and advised everybody to be vaccinated or re-vaccinated. Some doubt was expressed as to whether those who signed were involved in Gloucester general practice or even worked in the area.

The June statement confirmed that at that time no patients had been admitted to the new facility but it was ready and equipped. No deaths due to 'smallpox' had been reported at this stage.

Further information given to the public on 26 June confirmed that 126 cases were admitted to Brockworth. From other areas the reports of smallpox in Gloucester were being challenged as to their accuracy considering that patients were not 'invalids' as such, there was no morbidity or permanent scarring and no mortality. The apparent sudden increase in cases seems to have been due to the interference of the ministry officials. Two sanitary officers were appointed from elsewhere to help in managing diagnosis and isolation. Patients with any type of rash or pimple were at risk of being isolated. The authorities authorised ordering of more bedding and 12 children's cots were brought from the Children's Hospital. As the numbers of cases increased, permission was granted to extend the Brockworth facility with two additional blocks. Hadwen tried to settle the diagnosis as he was aware of a six-week-old baby that had been certified as dying of 'confluent smallpox'. He gained permission from the father for the coffin to be opened so that the body could be inspected to confirm the diagnosis. This was deemed unlawful and further investigation ceased.

Crisis of management arose over differing opinions and Dr Bibby was 'deposed' and replaced by Dr William Davidson from Birmingham. Dr Davidson's experience of smallpox was severely limited and therefore accuracy of diagnosis was doubted. The disagreement over true diagnosis had produced a division of opinions and Dr Bibby had re-emphasised his view that the main problem was chickenpox. There was further disquiet when Dr Davidson found that patients had been discharged from hospital without his concurrence. He was finding it impossible to keep track of patients' progress. Dr Davidson threatened resignation and at the same time the Matron resigned. The latter was replaced by a Miss Parnaby who was recently Matron of Hastings Borough Sanatorium at a salary of £5 per week. Two extra doctors with relevant experience were brought in to assist Dr Davidson, one with prime responsibility for the running of the Brockworth Unit. Their salary was fixed at £17 17s a week plus travelling expenses!

Dr Davidson further reported that 3,665 citizens were vaccinated between 8 June and 6 July. Employers also threatened that employees who refused vaccination would be given a week's notice and leave employment, even ex-servicemen working for the company, who may or may not have been vaccinated, were told to comply.

Before the meeting of the Health Committee on 27 June, Hadwen had left copies of an article at a councillor's house containing comments which criticised Dr Davidson and his surety of diagnosis. The meeting heard that the Medical Officer of Health for Bristol stated that from his experience, 'there is not the slightest shadow of doubt that this is smallpox'. One councillor, after visiting Brockworth, claimed there was a mix of both the mild and more severe type of smallpox under observation. The committee decided that, due to the confusion and uncertainty of diagnosis, an agreed experienced external Medical Officer, Dr Millard from Leicester. should make a thorough assessment. He arrived and examined the mild and severe cases and concluded that these were cases of smallpox. Hadwen stated:'The sole responsibility for all this horrible expense at Brockworth, a small fortune on taxi-cabs and conveyancing, all this despotism, these serious mistakes in diagnosis and the spuming of practical experience, rests with the Corporation of Gloucester'. Dr Davidson was assured of the full support of the Committee.

The Health Committee of the city council ruled that local medical practitioners could visit the hospital at any time but they must be accompanied by a Medical Officer of Health. The poor people of the city with the Co-operative Movement, their Unions and the Labour Party continued to support Hadwen's view that these diseases kept recurring in the city due to poor housing, poor sanitation and overcrowding. There was a policy of disinfecting houses where a family member had been diagnosed as a smallpox case and some householders refused for this to happen.

[Copy Report of Dr. Painton, referred to in Minute 1738.]

July, 1923.

To the Chairman and Members
   of the Health Committee.

THE EPIDEMIC OF *MILD* SMALLPOX IN GLOUCESTER.

The patients in the Brockworth Hospital have been seen by a large number of Medical Officers of Health, many of whom have had a very large experience with Smallpox for several years past, and the Public Health Department of Gloucester is authorised by the undermentioned Medical Officers to say that all the cases that have been seen in the Brockworth Hospital are cases of genuine Smallpox.

The letters written by these Medical Officers of Health on the subject may be seen at any time at the Health Office, 9, New Inn Lane, Gloucester, by anyone who wishes to verify the above statement.

One of the Medical Officers of Health of the largest Port in the United Kingdom writes as follows:—

"I take this occasion to state that, after an experience of over 20 years as Assistant Medical Officer of Health of this City and Port, and with extensive acquaintance with Smallpox both in this country and abroad, in addition to having seen the majority of the cases here during the epidemic of 1902-4, the diagnosis of the cases which I saw in the Brockworth Hospital was never for a moment in doubt in my mind. They were all genuine cases of Smallpox of a mild type, and not Chickenpox, Flea bites, Water rash, or Red Gum as has been stated. You may make what use you desire of this letter."

ADVERTISEMENT.

To the Citizens of Gloucester Parents & Employees

Dr. HADWEN'S reply to the speeches and to the attack made upon him personally at the Council Meeting on Wednesday last has been refused publication by the Editor of the Citizen. It will therefore be published otherwise, circulated and distributed to every house in Gloucester.

A Protest Meeting

WILL BE HELD AT THE

TABERNACLE, DERBY ROAD

ON

Wednesday next, June 27th 1923

At 7.30 p.m.

Chairman : E. H. SPRING, Esq.

The Meeting will be addressed by

Dr. Walter R. Hadwen

AND OTHERS.

Come and Protest.

Printed by Gloucester Printers, Ltd., Hopewell Street.
Published by The (P. G. Eastwood-Robinson) Service, 6, Southgate St., for Walter R. Hadwen, 35, Brunswick Square.

Force was sometimes used to effect isolation and objection was expressed as some people felt that the law was being misinterpreted. In August, a father was charged at the city Petty Sessions of unlawfully obstructing the execution of the order to remove his child, Winnie Smith, as a medical certificate stated that she was 'suffering from a dangerous infectious disorder, to wit, smallpox' the household accommodation in which they lived could not provide a suitable facility for isolation of the case. The father pleaded guilty, Hadwen was in Court at first observing. It was admitted that the epidemic was almost over and by the time the case came to court the child was deemed to be over the period of infectiousness. The standard penalty for refusal to comply was ten pounds and it was stated that a sanitary inspector had attended the household along with a police constable to enforce the Magistrate's order. The Court decided that the charge was 'obstruction' at which point Hadwen arose and requested permission to say a few words. The Bench decided no good would be done by him addressing the Magistrates and Hadwen admitted that they had no alternative to conviction. The assistant solicitor to the Gloucester Corporation objected to Hadwen being allowed to say more. Hadwen persisted that there were a few observations he wished to make and also to put in an appeal on behalf of the defendant. He was allowed to continue and asked the Bench for permission to show that the basis on which the order had been made was not justifiable. After further legal wrangling and debate over the bad wording of the act, Hadwen was asked to limit his remarks to the character of the defendant. Hadwen went on and stated that there was sufficient accommodation in the defendant's house and there were two rooms available that had never been used and the father had stated that the house had not been inspected. The magistrate who signed the order did not see the rooms, neither had the Sanitary Inspector. The inspecting doctor saw the rooms and he commented he was convinced that this was not a dangerous infective disease but a mild form of chickenpox. The law appeared to be at least open to interpretation! He would make the case for the defendant. The father could not afford the fine and he hoped a heavy fine would not be inflicted. If they did the defendant would be compelled to go to prison. The defendant loved his child more than he loved himself. Further legal arguments took place. The fine was set at £5 and the defendant given a month to pay. Later Hadwen went to the Police Station and paid the fine himself, on behalf of Mr Smith.

By all accounts the effectiveness of 'isolation' was poorly supervised. The attempt to keep patients within the barbed wire fence boundary was not foolproof and ways were soon found to meet up and mix with visiting friends and family. Family picnics together were known to occur at weekends. The local population called the Brockworth Isolation Unit 'Pimple Town'. A Councillor had donated several cricket sets so the patients could amuse themselves whilst waiting permission to be discharged. The number of 'patients' under observation there was averaging about 100. Exaggerations of the 'epidemic' affected trade in the city but locally it was felt that this minor disease did not even justify the closing of schools.

Many in the local population treated it as a bit of a joke. The 'patients' were not ill, had a vague rash and none was bed bound. Far from it, the Matron wrote a letter stating that the 'patients enjoyed themselves playing in the grounds, playing tennis and other games'. Three deaths were attributed to smallpox but this figure was thrown into doubt as those who died had other medical conditions which were far more likely to have caused their demise. The peak of cases by July in isolation was 254. By the end of August cases had markedly declined. Later in 1923 there was a city Council election and Dr Bibby was elected to serve.

The Bishop, Dr. Headlam, declared this to be 'Divine judgement' and prayed for 'succour in this time of distress', fuelling the idea that the epidemic was far more serious than was justified, and urging that it was everyone's duty to be vaccinated and the scourge could be stamped out. He composed a letter to be read to all the city congregations, dated 30 June. He stated how city trade had been badly affected and the cost and heavy expenses of the Public Health services would affect the rates. Science was not infallible but it has accomplished a lot and we must avail ourselves of that knowledge to conquer this medical problem. He specifically mentions the consequences of bad housing and unsanitary conditions. There needed to be a spirit of fairness and not blame. The situation required a spirit of wisdom and understanding.

This letter was formulated without him personally assessing the reality of the situation. He appointed another priest to visit Brockworth who, like every visitor, had to prove recent vaccination and should wear overalls provided.

7 Old Tram Rd
Albion St
June 28. 1923

Dear Tom & Ada
just a few lines to let you know we are keeping allright hoping you are the same. we have not Smallpox in Gloster. I dont even beleive its catching whatever it is they reckon we have had it in Gloster over 6 months. now you dont want anything plainer than that. not one death that speaks for itself. you will find enclosed two bills from Dr Hadwen the papers would not print his letters. so he had bills printed & sent round. read them well & form your own opinion of them. I had a little chat with the Dr on Sunday he told me then it was not what they said it was. I came across a cutting out of the Citizen printed 1883 that is 40 years ago relating to Smallpox 46 ago that makes it 86 years. it was a cure for Smallpox someone took a copy of it and sent it to the paper but they have not printed it. I am sending the cure for you. I am so sorry for Lizzie Remember us to all I remain
Yours Ted

7, Old Tram Rd, Albion St
June 28. 1923

Dear Tom and Ada,
just a few lines to let you know we are keeping alright hoping you are the same. we have not smallpox in Gloster, I don't even believe its they reckon we have had it in Gloster over 6 months. now you don't want anything plainer than that. not one death that speaks for itself. you will find enclosed two bills from Dr Hadwen. The papers would not print his letters, so he had bills printed & sent round. read them well and form your own opinion of them. I had a little chat with the Dr on Sunday he told then it was not what they said it was. I came across a cutting out of the Citizen printed 1883 that is 40 years ago relating to smallpox 46 years ago that makes it 86 years it was a cure for smallpox. someone took a copy of it and sent it to the paper but they have not printed it. I am sending the cure for you. I am so sorry for Lizzy, Remember us to all. I remain, Yours, Ted

Hadwen commented on this unnecessary scaremongering. Owners of seaside lodgings were induced by the press to refuse hospitality to Gloucester holiday-makers. The Mayor visited the Brockworth hospital on the 25th July but his report to the council was hardly reassuring. The Matron wrote to the local press of the Mayor's visit and stated there were only six patients in bed but were there for unrelated diagnoses. She stated she had seen 144 cases admitted and not one could be described as 'severe' or 'ghastly' as stated by the Mayor and all were 'quite well' on admission with a few papules, vesicles or pustules. Hadwen himself overrated his opinion that smallpox was not as dangerous as measles or scarlet fever, if treated correctly by baths and oil. In fact his letter in the local *Citizen* paper stated that there was a great risk to vaccination, it may ruin a child's life and diseased hundreds of thousands and caused the death of a great number. He believed that within a few years the practice of vaccination would be punishable by law.

10
REX V HADWEN
OCTOBER 27TH, 28TH, 29TH, 1924

FIRSTLY, it was a rarity for a Doctor to be accused of manslaughter and the circumstances have been described in reports and articles in the newspapers of the day. Much interpretation has been made of whether there was a vendetta carried out by the local members of the medical profession. There was jealousy as regards Hadwen's popularity amongst his patients and it is said that not one patient left his practice during the events surrounding his trial. There was animosity by the profession against his dogmatic views of opposition to vaccination and immunisation as a treatment and also his fight against animal cruelty and vivisection. The BUAV produced a 60 page booklet which presented a verbatim report on the actual trial and included additional comments from those who supported Hadwen's views. Ten thousand copies of this booklet were printed priced one shilling. (I have three copies). There are some preliminary comments quoting correspondence between Dr Ellis and Dr Hadwen demonstrating some ill feeling that had arisen before the trial and Hadwen's attempt to reconcile opposing opinions.

To understand the circumstances of the trial I have reproduced the report of the inquest held at Gloucester petty sessions in Appendix 1. This was held in the court where Hadwen had served as magistrate. This coroners court was set up in September 1924 to investigate the circumstances of the death of Nellie Burnham on 10 August 1924. I feel that it is very important to understand in detail each step of this hearing and subsequent trial, and to explain how this all affected Hadwen. Hadwen's life story would be incomplete without a full insight into what happened.

After hearing evidence for seven hours the jury, at the inquest, pronounced a verdict 'that the child died from diphtheria and pneumonia and that Dr Hadwen failed to show competent skill and special attention, in consequence of which failure the child died'. The jury took three quarters of an hour to reach the verdict which the foreman stated was the verdict of nine of the twelve jurymen.

The coroner then pronounced that in law this was a verdict of manslaughter, and therefore there must be a verdict accordingly. There must be a committal, whereupon he instructed Dr Hadwen to stand and stated that he had no alternative but 'to commit you on my inquisition to take your trial at the next Assizes for the city of Gloucester'. Bail was arranged. He was told to report to the Police Station the following Saturday. Despite this setback, Hadwen maintained his dignity and continued with his practice consultations, his preaching and his regular session as a magistrate.

The interval between the Coroner's inquest and the trial for manslaughter must have been a very stressful time for him and family, but he had an inner conviction that all would turn out well and that he had the support of the public as well as experienced members of the legal profession to advise him.

I have made the decision to record as accurate a summary of this important trial by using the report from the *British Medical Journal*. An audio-tape was produced in the 1990s featuring Edgar Lustgarten, a famous barrister and author with a re-enactment of the trial as interpreted and presented in dramatic fashion by Lustgarten himself.

A report as a synopsis of the Trial on a charge of manslaughter at Gloucester assizes, published in the *British Medical Journal*

The trial of Dr W. R. Hadwen of Gloucester, on an indictment for manslaughter arising out of the death of a child whom he had attended, took place at Gloucester Assizes on October 27th, 28th and 29th before Mr Justice Lush. The counsel in the case were Mr C. F. Vachell. K. C. and Mr St. John G. Micklethwait, on behalf of the Director of Public Prosecutions, and Sir E. Marshall-Hall, K. C. and Mr A. F. Clements for the defence.

Dr Hadwen pleaded "Not Guilty".

The charge was " Walter Hadwen, you are charged for that you, at the Parish of Gloucester, on the 10th day of August, 1924, did feloniously kill and slay one Nellie Burnham, against the Peace".

Case for the Prosecution.
Mr Vachell, in opening the case, said that Nellie Burnham, aged 10, died on August 10th last from diphtheria and pneumonia which followed it. She was attended in her illness by Dr Hadwen who, the prosecution alleged, failed, through gross inattention and lack of skill or knowledge, or both, to detect the disease from which the child was suffering and to administer the proper remedy. Counsel then described the common symptoms of diphtheria and the general procedure of the medical profession in such cases, more particularly the taking of a swab from the patient's throat and the administration of antitoxin. He went on to review at length the circumstances of the case, and said that, in spite of the highly suspicious symptoms, Dr Hadwen never took a swab from the throat or administered antitoxin. A fact to which, he understood, the defence attached importance was that two days before her death, while the mother was away from home, the child left her bed and went barefooted downstairs into the scullery to get a drink of water, but the evidence to be called with regard to the post-mortem examination would show that the pneumonia was of a type which followed diphtheria, and not of the type that followed a chill.

Mrs Burnham said that her daughter was taken ill on July 30th, and Dr. Hadwen, her club doctor, was called in on August 1st. He remarked that the case looked like scarlet fever. He put two fingers in the girl's mouth and examined her throat and examined her back and chest for any rash. He prescribed a gargle of vinegar and water. His examination occupied only three minutes. The breath was very offensive, and there was a yellowish discharge tinged with blood from the nose. She mentioned the foulness of breath to the doctor on his second visit on August 4th, when he looked down the child's throat, using his finger as before, but did not feel her pulse or take her temperature. He came next on August 6th, by which time she was weaker and the breath more offensive. By this time the nose had a yellowish, spongy appearance like the throat. The doctor's next visit was on August 9th, when, the child being weaker, she sent for him. He looked down the throat, felt the pulse, and sounded the chest, but did not take her temperature. He said that the throat was clearing nicely. He stayed about 5 minutes. At the previous visit he had prescribed a tonic. He did not take a swab at any time. The child vomited first on August 8th. On the evening of August 9th, the child being evidently worse, there was a family consultation, and

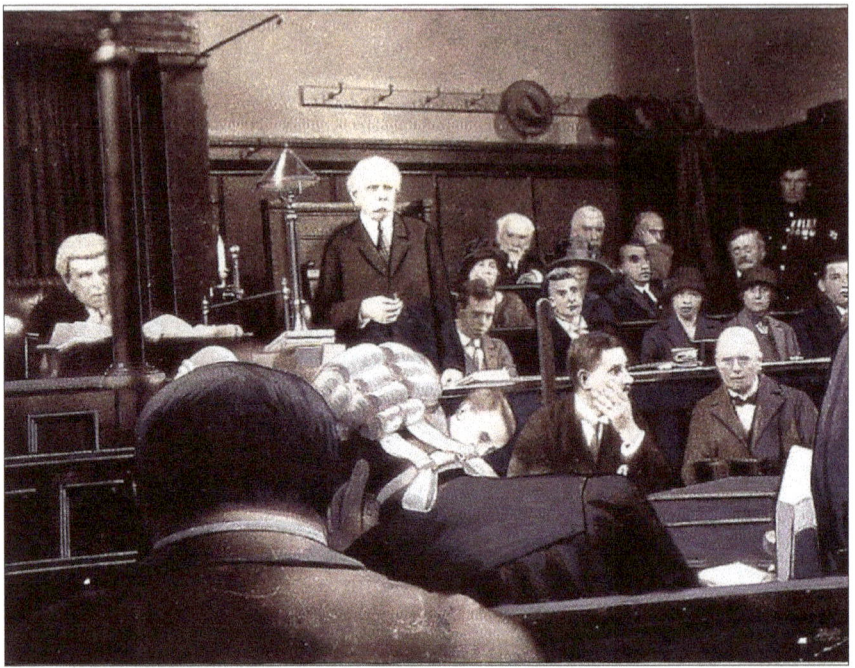

Court scenes from the trial of Dr Hadwen, October 1924

Dr Ellis was summoned. He took a swab of the throat, and examined the child's chest and back, but she was then in a very grave state, and died on the early morning of the 10th.

In cross examination certain discrepancies in the evidence given by the witness compared with the evidence she gave at the coroner's court were pointed out: these related to the date on which she first suspected the case to be of diphtheria. In reply to further questions, she said that she sent for Dr Ellis on the recommendation of her brother-in-law. She knew nothing of an acrimonious dispute between Dr. Ellis and Dr Hadwen in the public press. She did not tell Dr Ellis that Dr Hadwen had seen the child earlier that day, but he was informed that Dr Hadwen had been attending the case and was told what Dr Hadwen had done. Dr Ellis was willing to give a death certificate, but she did not wish for one, because, being dissatisfied with Dr Hadwen's treatment, she wanted to have an inquest. It had not occurred to her that it was not quite fair to Dr Hadwen not to tell him that the child was dead, so that he might be present at the post-mortem examination. She admitted that it was a rule of her society that in an emergency patients might send for the doctor at any time, and that she did not send for Dr Hadwen after his visit on the 6th until the morning of the 9th, but she thought 'it was his place

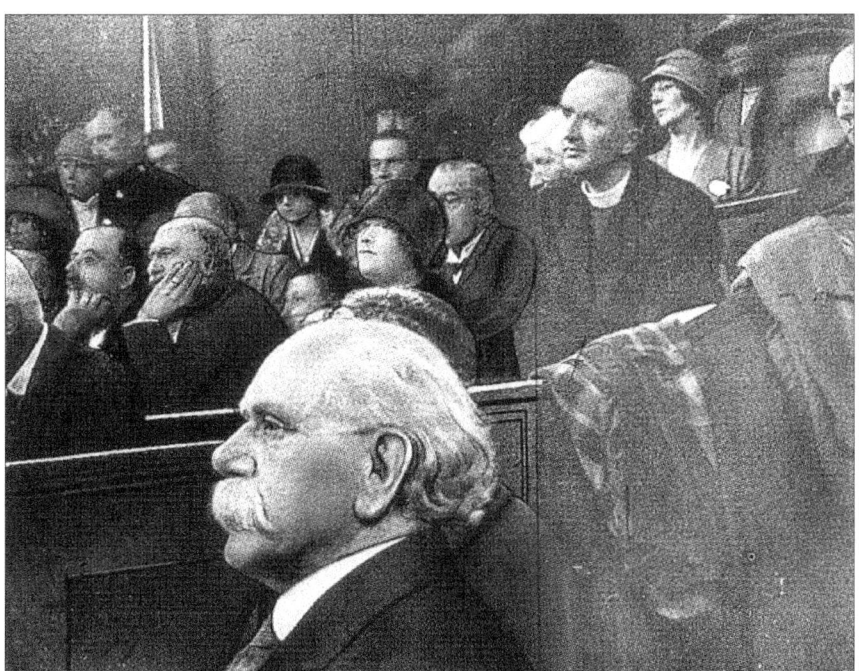

to come without being sent for every time'. His Lordship asked whether, when the doctor came two days after the child had been downstairs, she told him of that incident, the witness replied that she did not. Re-examined, she said that when Dr Ellis was called in, three hours before the child died, it was the first time she had ever seen him. He stayed two hours, he showed no ill feeling towards Dr Hadwen, and said nothing about Dr. Hadwen's treatment.

Other witnesses — members of the family and neighbours — were called and gave similar evidence. A brother-in-law of Mrs Burnham said that, late on the evening before the child's death, he, as a result of a family counsel telephoned Dr. Hadwen to the effect that they were not satisfied with his treatment and had decided to call in another doctor. Dr. Hadwen had replied that he had done his best. Dr. Ellis had been the witness's own doctor.

Dr E. S. Ellis said that when called to attend the child he found her seriously ill with a temperature of 102.5 degrees and a pulse rate of 154. Her general condition was toxaemic. When he came he was told that it was probably a case of diphtheria. He noticed her very rapid breathing, and at once thought of pneumonia. He found the right lung solid and the left bronchitic. In the throat he found membrane right across from tonsil to tonsil. There was a discharge from one nostril, a greenish dirty discharge, just tinged with blood. He took a swab, and then he wondered whether there might not be fluid in the chest, but on exploration found no pneumonia. He had no doubt whatsoever as to the diphtheria even before the result of the examination of the swab was available, and he notified it at once, there was such obvious diphtheritic membrane. He did not administer anti-toxin because it was too late, the child was dying.

In the course of a long cross-examination by Sir E. Marshall-Hall, Dr. Ellis expressed the opinion that the diphtheria spread down into the lung: it was really all one disease. The pneumonia in this case was unilateral according to the post-mortem findings.

Have you ever known a case of pneumonia, the sequel of diphtheria, which has been unilateral?

Witness:- No, nor bilateral either.

Must it not be one or the other

Witness:- I have never come across a case before, the cases go to the hospital. It is a question for the pathologist.

Was pneumonia in this case lobar or lobular?

Witness: When I auscultated that chest it was so late the whole thing was solid, it might have been either.

At a later stage in the cross examination counsel asked the witness whether, in August, 1923, he wrote to the editors of two London daily papers inviting them to send representatives to interview him with reference to Dr. Hadwen, and whether in the course of his communication, which was not printed, he made a violent attack on Dr Hadwen and his professional status? Dr Ellis said there was certainly communication, and he had pointed out a discrepancy between Dr Hadwen's qualifications as given in the medical Register and in a book printed locally. There had been a very acrimonious correspondence in the local press between himself and Dr. Hadwen over the vaccination question. Later he was asked for information by the London newspapers and a reporter called upon him. Dr. Hadwen had been communicating to the public press matters derogatory to the witness and everybody else in the profession, he suggested that the epidemic at Gloucester was not smallpox but chickenpox, and that the whole epidemic had been trumped up for the benefit of the doctors.

Re-examined by Mr Vachell, Dr. Ellis said that the epidemic in Gloucester was of smallpox, with a certain amount of chickenpox. Dr Hadwen wrote a letter, inserting it as an advertisement in the local press, dealing with this subject from the anti-vaccination point of view. The witness entered into some private correspondence with Dr. Hadwen on the matter and was afterwards asked by 3 reporters for some information. At about the time this case arose there were some overtures with a view to making up the differences between the medical men in Gloucester.

Dr. W. Washbourn, city bacteriologist, who made the postmortem examination, described his findings. The back of the throat, tonsils, soft palate, and larynx were intensely inflamed, almost black in one or two places. An adherent patch of membrane at the back of the epiglottis was characteristic of diphtheria. Both bronchial tubes were congested. the right bronchial tubes were filled with dense membrane, some of which was adherent and had evidently been formed in situ. At the top of the bronchus was a piece of diphtheritic membrane, measuring about 3 inches by one inch. In the pleural cavity there was a small quantity of fluid-about three ounces. He could give an opinion with confidence as to the cause of death. It was due to diphtheria and pneumonia. He found the diphtheria bacillus present in the swab received on the day of the girl's death. He received other swabs a day or two later from the medical officer of the isolation hospital. He learned afterwards that these were taken from members of the family of the dead girl and a playmate. Two were negative and two were positive.

In cross-examination the witness expressed the opinion that the condition of the right lung was that of lobar pneumonia of recent date—not more than two or three days old. When he examined the swab he was not aware that the child from whom it had been taken was dead. Although the Klebs-Loeffler bacillus was recognised by the great majority of the profession to be the specific bacillus of diphtheria, it could be found also in some cases where there was no diphtheria. He was aware, just before starting the postmortem examination, that the child had been Dr. Hadwen's patient, and that there was some charge of negligence against Dr. Hadwen in his treatment of the case. Dr Bell, Deputy Coroner (then acting-coroner), was present at the examination, not at his invitation but as a right, and he (witness) asked him whether Dr. Hadwen was going to be present. He thought the deputy coroner answered that Dr Hadwen had been invited or that he was not coming. After referring to further questions, mainly about the symptoms of diphtheria and pneumonia, the witness said that the membrane he found at postmortem was undoubtedly diphtheritic, but he did not examine it microscopically, he thought it so clear that it was not necessary to examine further. Later the witness said that in this case, so far as he could judge, the heart was healthy. In a great many cases, but by no means in all, fatty degeneration would accompany acute diphtheria.

The duration of the pneumonia found postmortem would fit in, although a 'tight fit', with the theory that the pneumonia was set up when the child, two nights before her death, got out of bed and went downstairs. He did not think pneumonia caused by such a chill would have begun to manifest itself until 12 to 24 hours afterwards, but it was impossible to eliminate the circumstances as a cause of pneumonia. Nevertheless, he felt sure that the diphtheria was a very large determining factor in the death of the child; the right bronchial tubes were also extensively involved in membrane that this would have been likely to set up right sided pneumonia.

Dr R. B. Berry, M. O. H. for Gloucester and medical superintendent of the city isolation hospital, described the proper course to take when a doctor found the familiar symptoms of diphtheria present. He spoke of members of the Burnham family who had been admitted to the isolation hospital during August suffering from diphtheria. In cross examination, he admitted that the antitoxin treatment was not always successful. He considered the pneumonia in this case was secondary to the diphtheria. The child died from the diphtheria progressing through pneumonia to death.

Dr E Graham of Gloucester said that he attended, as per panel doctor, an elder sister of Nellie Burnham on the day after the girl's death. He took a swab of the throat and sent it to the Medical Officer of Health. In cross-examination he acknowledged himself a strong opponent of Dr. Hadwen.

Sir William Willcox, in reply to Mr Vachell, gave a description of diphtheria, its origin and symptoms. Vomiting might occur at the onset, and again at a later stage when the disease became dangerous. It was a grave sign after the first or second day. He outlined the prudent course for a medical man to take on finding a patient suffering from sore throat, thickness of utterance, offensive breath, coloured discharge from the nose, and drowsiness. A swab should be taken, and if there was to the naked eye a reasonable suspicion of diphtheria, as evidenced by visible membrane or patches of exudate in the throat, then it would be his duty to give antitoxin without waiting for the result of bacteriological examination. Diphtheria antitoxin had reduced the mortality of diphtheria from 30 or 40 per cent, down to 10 per cent, and under. In 1893, two years before the antitoxin treatment was first used in this country, the mortality from diphtheria was 389 per million in England and Wales; the figure in 1923 was 71 per million. In his judgement the cause of this child's death was diphtheria and pneumonia. Hearing the evidence he had no doubt the pneumonia was secondary to the diphtheria. It was uncommon for this kind of pneumonia to be unilateral, but he had seen it occur in diphtheria. It was very difficult to say whether this was lobar or lobular; but in view of the condition of the right bronchial tubes he thought this was a massive or very extensive bronchopneumonia. In his opinion this child's journey downstairs would not cause the pneumonia such as was found in this case, though it would, of course, be harmful at that stage of the disease and would subject the child to grave risk of heart failure. In further evidence the witness said that Dr Ellis did quite the right thing in using the exploratory needle two hours before death. It was difficult in children from clinical examination to be certain whether there was solid lung or fluid. The risk in using the needle was infinitesimal. In diphtheria the only treatment of any value was antitoxin treatment with general hygienic care. Supposing the pneumonia was independent of the diphtheria, the fact that the child was already suffering from the neglected diphtheria would greatly diminish the resistance to the pneumonia, however caused.

Sir William Wilcox, in cross-examination, said he saw quite a number of early cases of diphtheria in his hospital practice. A long argument then ensued on the figures in the Registrar-General's returns which, counsel contended, did not bear out the statement that the diphtheria was now a less deadly disease than formerly.

The witness explained the meaning or the categories and the significance of the figures under each heading, and repeated that there had been a steady decline in the death rate from the disease: in 1895 it was 313 per million of the population and it was now 71. Counsel next referred to statistics for 1922, which showed that 2, 021 cases wrongly diagnosed as diphtheria had been admitted to the Metropolitan Asylums Board hospitals, and that of these patients 77 had died.

Witness pointed out that these figures were for the London fever hospitals, that the poorer districts of London were much more overcrowded, and that there was a tendency for practitioners to send cases to hospital when at all suspicious of diphtheria, without waiting for the result of a swab, lest other inmates of the crowded dwelling became infected. These 'wrong diagnoses' were cases of bad throats in which diphtheria was suspected but the bacteriological examination proved negative. If these 'mistakes' were not made the amount of diphtheria in London would be much greater. Counsel next quoted from Sir George Newman's report for 1921, in which he referred to the figures for diphtheria due to the notification as diphtheria of cases of mild illness which seldom presented any definite clinical evidence and would not be regarded as cases of this disease apart from the fact of contact or the receipt of a positive report on throat swabs.

Witness said that this was true; some doctors were over-cautious and notified diphtheria when the signs were by no means conclusive. Counsel asked why the same argument should not apply to the Registrar-General's returns. Witness pointed out that these returns were based simply on death certificates. He was next cross-examined on Dr. Washbourn's account of the postmortem findings. In reply to the judge, he gave a brief account of the nature and preparation of antitoxins and vaccines, and was questioned as to the doctor's duty if he went counter to the opinion of the vast majority of his profession.

At the close of these questions his lordship addressing Sir Edward Marshall-Hall, said "You are faced with this difficulty, Sir Edward, that a person may hold a bona fide belief in some remedy without calling in a doctor at all, but the courts have held that an honest belief that the doctors do no good, and that prayers alone have efficacy, does not dispose of wilful neglect for not calling in a doctor. The Legislature compels a parent to call a doctor into his child.

Counsel: But no Legislature has yet compelled a doctor to inoculate with anti-diphtheritic serum.

His Lordship: No; but the difficulty still remains which I have pointed out.

Counsel next produced a work on differential diagnosis, and asked whether, in view of the diagrams in that book, the diagnosis between follicular tonsillitis and diphtheria might be very difficult.

Witness said that it might be impossible unless a swab was taken. Asked whether there was no real danger in inoculating a patient who had previously been inoculated with serum, he said that he had never seen any real fatal case through the use of anti-diphtheritic serum. If a patient had had serum previously the second dose was given with special precautions. After further questions by counsel for the defence, and a short re-examination by Mr Vachell, his worship asked Sir William Wilcox a number of questions about the efficacy of diphtheria antitoxin generally, and its efficiency when given early or late in the disease.

Case for the defence
Dr Hadwen, giving evidence in his own behalf stated his qualifications, M. D. St. Andrews, L. R. C. P. Lond. , M. R. C. S. Eng. , L. M. S. S. A. He said he had practised for over 30 years. He had had a fair amount of experience of diphtheria, and about 25 years ago was practising in Bristol when an epidemic of diphtheria occurred, and most of the cases were under his care.

He had never administered antitoxin, and all his cases had been successful. Dr. Hadwen then described his treatment of the dead child's brother Leonard, who was suffering from septic tonsillitis. He suspected diphtheria in Leonard's case, and satisfied himself absolutely that no diphtheria was there. He next attended another child of the same family, who had the infection in a lighter degree. When first called to Nellie, she had been ill for two days. He examined the throat and found three ulcerative spots on the right tonsil, two on the left, the throat was red. He found no rash, but there was a little watery discharge from the nose. He found a little harsh breathing in the chest, pointing to slight bronchial catarrh. He ordered an expectorant mixture and a gargle of vinegar and hot water, and gave a few general directions. He felt the child's pulse as a matter of course on every visit. The pulse was quicker than normal and the temperature 100 degrees. His visit lasted roughly ten minutes. The child was a poorly nourished, ill conditioned girl. He saw no yellow, blood-streaked discharge, nor detected any offensive breath, and the mother never said a word to him about such things. At his visits on August 4th and 5th the throat was better, the bronchial catarrh had cleared up, and the child was much better. He intended to go again on the 9th but was too busy, he was on his way there on the 9th when he was sent for. He was thunderstruck at the change in the child, and saw at once that her condition was serious. The throat had cleared up nicely, there was not a single vestige of ulceration on the tonsil, there was no membrane either upon the uvula or soft palate. The breath sounds were reduced, temperature 101 degrees, pulse 120, he concluded. The mother never told him that the child had been downstairs. He intended to call again that night, but was informed by telephone that the family had called in another doctor. He heard of the child's death about an hour before the inquest was held. He had no notice of the postmortem examination. He reaffirmed his opinion that the child had been suffering from ulcerative or septic tonsillitis, and that she developed fatal lobar pneumonia.

In cross-examination by Mr Vachell, Dr. Hadwen said that he had doubted whether during the last three years he had any cases of diphtheria at all. To administer antitoxin was against his views and his conscience, he considered it a very dangerous remedy. All these inoculations were based upon experiments on animals, he objected to them on that ground, but he objected to the antitoxin independently as a medical man. He was taken by counsel through the usual symptoms of diphtheria and their relative importance, and questioned by the judge on antitoxin. A long discussion then ensued between his lordship, counsel and witness on the Registrar-General's statistics. Dr. Hadwen went on to say that he believed the bacillus to be the result of disease, not its cause, and he saw no sense in taking a swab. He discarded the whole germ theory of disease. Asked by the judge what was his theory of the communication of disease, he spoke of a chemical poison in the atmosphere. The specific cause could not be discovered, but insanitary conditions affecting the atmosphere produced the disease. Asked what would have been the treatment had he found diphtheria, he said he would have put hot fomentations around the throat, painted the tonsils with glycerine three or four times a day, and cautioned the mother to keep the child in a recumbent position. He would, of course, have notified the case, and in the circumstances would have the child's removal to the isolation hospital. He contested Dr Washbourn's opinion that the membrane he found was diphtheritic.

In re-examination by his counsel, Dr. Hadwen returned to the question of statistics. He said that with the introduction of antitoxin, diphtheria, instead of being diagnosed in the old fashioned way, became diagnosed by a very different method, with the result that a great many common sore throats, which would have got well in any circumstances, were called diphtheria, and this had led to an apparent decrease in mortality.

Speeches of Counsel
Mr Vachell then addressed the jury at some length, recapitulating the evidence which had been offered on behalf of the prosecution. He made a strong point of the fact that no medical evidence other than Dr. Hadwen's had been called by the defence. Sir E Marshall-Hall followed with a speech of much greater length for the defence. He strongly attacked the credibility of one of the witnesses who had altered her evidence as to what she saw of the sick child, she had said one thing in the earlier

proceedings and quite a different thing in the present trial after having in the meantime heard the medical evidence. He also described it as most unfortunate that the second doctor called in by the family in this case was one who had been a most bitter opponent of Dr. Hadwen in the press. Dr Ellis never communicated the fact of the child's death to Dr. Hadwen, and what was still worse, the deputy-coroner (Dr. Bell) gave no notice of the postmortem examination to the man against whom, on the result of the examination, it was intended to prefer a charge. Counsel hoped it would not be inferred that Dr. Hadwen was the only medical man in England opposed to the administration of antitoxin. He could not afford to keep eminent specialists at the court for three or four days.

The Judge's Summing-up
Mr Justice Lush, at the beginning of his charge to the jury, said that the case was a serious one, with consequences to others than the immediate defendant.

It is a matter of great importance also to the public, and, I may say to the medical profession, because while, on the one hand, persons are entitled to be and must be, protected against criminal neglect or criminal misconduct on the part of a medical man, it would be deplorable, disastrous, if a medical man, following his profession according to the best of his judgement and acting honestly in the treatment of his patient, were to have hanging over his head a fear that if anything went wrong with his patient there might be a prosecution such as this.

It was a case also which called for strong and clear proof on the part of the Crown. The jury was not sitting merely to criticise Dr. Hadwen's views. It was not a case merely of saying whether he had or had not adopted views which a wise medical man should have adopted. The charge against him was that he 'did feloniously kill' the child, and it was necessary for the Crown to establish, not only that he neglected her, but that his neglect did actually cause her death. Many cases had been tried in which a medical man, qualified or unqualified, had, in endeavouring to cure a patient, chosen to administer a dangerous drug or perform some operation, and if the drug was administered or the operation performed in a disgraceful and careless fashion, or with a disgraceful ignorance as to what the effect of the drug would be or as to the way in which the operation should have been performed, and the patient died, there was no difficulty in saying that the doctor or operator caused the death of the patient. What was said in this case was very different. It was that Dr Hadwen was so neglectful in his diagnosis and treatment that the child, whose life would have been saved if proper care had been taken, died through that neglect.

If a doctor is culpably negligent in his treatment of a patient, and the patient dies, it is not enough for the Crown in supporting an indictment of manslaughter, to prove that if the doctor had been careful, the patient would have had a chance of getting successfully through the illness. The Crown must prove more than that, they must prove that in all human probability, if care had been used the child would have recovered. If the Crown have established to your reasonable satisfaction, first that the doctor did neglect the child, and secondly that in all human probability the child would have recovered if he had not neglected her then, and then only, you will bring a verdict of 'Guilty'.

His lordship considered that August 1st, the date on which Dr Hadwen first saw the patient, was the important date in the case. The doctor had already attended the child's brother for a similar illness, and the boy had recovered. When he was called to see the child who subsequently died he found her not as bad as her brother had been, and although he had called on the brother every day he did not call on the girl again until after three days. Did the child on the first visit show such signs as would make an ordinary doctor suspect diphtheria, or did she only show the signs of sore throat?

Sir William Wilcox had stated that unless antitoxin was given within six days from the commencement of the illness it was practically useless, and if Dr. Hadwen had no reason on his first visit to suspect anything seriously wrong with the child's throat, the child having already been ill for two days, any neglect of the child from the second visit onwards would not make the with-holding of the antitoxin a matter of very serious importance. The Crown had to prove to the reasonable satisfaction of the jury that on the first visit the child showed signs of a serious malady which the doctor refused to consider.

Next came the question of the pneumonia. If the pneumonia was really a sequel of diphtheria, then supposing the doctor to be responsible for the diphtheritic condition, he was equally responsible for the pneumonia. But if the pneumonia was brought about by the unfortunate act on behalf of the child – going downstairs with bare feet on the tiled floor, which set up a chill, and the pneumonia caused death, no one could say that neglect on the part of the doctor in the early days of the case had anything to do with causing the death of the child.

I come now to the question of neglect. The law does not say that if a doctor is unfortunate enough to commit an error of judgement and the patient dies he is guilty of manslaughter. The law does not cast upon anybody who is merely careless, and whose carelessness is the cause of death of another, the responsibility of defending himself in the dock on this charge. Unless the negligence of which a person is guilty is of so gross a character as to make one say of it that it is wicked negligence, not a careless, but a wickedly careless thing to have done, the person concerned cannot be convicted of manslaughter.

There must be something evil in the negligence, something culpable, something criminal, before an indictment of manslaughter can be established. You have got to ask yourselves, not whether Dr Hadwen failed to exercise that care which a doctor or anybody else ought to exercise, but whether he was guilty of what I have called culpable and wicked negligence. If he was, then the Crown have proved the first of the two things they have to prove, if he was not, the Crown have failed to prove even the first step.

His Lordship then reviewed the evidence of the mother and her friends, reminding the jury that the mother's evidence as to the bad condition of the child on the first visit was uncorroborated. One could make all allowances for the mother, but she had not behaved in all aspects quite in the way one might have expected her to behave. She never told the doctor the very important circumstances of the child's visit to the kitchen, and the jury might come to the conclusion that the mother's evidence was exaggerated as to the condition of the child on August 1st. If the condition of the child was as Dr. Hadwen said it was, his Lordship could not conceive of any ground for considering him guilty of criminal negligence in not taking a swab. He next dwelt with the evidence relating to the second and subsequent visits of the doctor, and pointed out how the stories of the relatives and of the doctor conflicted.

Coming to the medical evidence his Lordship said that if the child never had diphtheria then away went the case for the prosecution. The child undoubtedly had pneumonia; if there was no diphtheria to cause the pneumonia it was probably caused by the chill. It did not follow that if it was proved that the child had diphtheria, the doctor was criminally neglectful, but here came the singular aspect of the case. Dr. Hadwen's views and mental attitude were different from those general in his profession. The jury was not a tribunal to criticise his views.

But I think it is legitimate to say that it would be very unfortunate if any doctor were to close his eyes to the improvements in medical treatment which were accepted by the great majority of his profession, and to say ' I prefer the old-fashioned treatment, I do not believe in these others'. After all, medical science is a very great science, and the medical profession a very great profession, and unless a doctor is going to avail himself of the discoveries made from time to time one is not likely to see that development of medical science which one hopes to see. It does not follow from that, of course, that a man who will stick to his own views is guilty of culpable and wicked neglect. A doctor, if properly qualified, is allowed by law to follow and practice his profession in the way he accepts, and if a doctor does hold peculiar views, honestly hold them, and works them out and follows them, one cannot say that there is any culpable and wicked neglect, even though he is terribly and seriously mistaken. But a doctor or anybody else, it is not for me to pass judgement on Dr Hadwen, may get his mind into such a state of prejudice and allow his judgement to be so blinded that really his position comes to this, that he would rather sacrifice his patient than sacrifice his prejudice. I do not say that is true of Dr. Hadwen at all, but there comes a stage when a man must be judged by what he does.

Was the child (continued his Lordship) suffering from diphtheria? The prosecution has got a very powerful body of evidence bearing on that question, the positive result of the swab, the coming away of the membrane, the positive results found in the two other children. Curiously enough, however, there was a very strong difference of opinion between Sir William Wilcox and Dr. Washbourn. Dr Washbourn's opinion, though it was only natural that, in deference to Sir William Willcox's views, he should not hold it quite so strongly as at first, was that the pneumonia which caused the death was lobar pneumonia, and that would be an indication, not of a secondary pneumonia brought on by diphtheria, but of a pneumonia caused by a chill. Sir William Willcox took the opposite view, and stated that the pneumonia must have been lobular and a sequel of diphtheria. It was for the Crown to prove that there was no reasonable doubt, and if the doubt still remained he would warn the jury that they must be very careful before they convicted the defendant of manslaughter. The neglect alleged against him was not in allowing the pneumonia to supervene, but in not discovering that there was diphtheria and taking proper steps. His Lordship added:

I cannot help saying that I agree with Sir E. Marshall-Hall that in a case like this, when this step, not often taken, of bringing a charge against a practising doctor in respect to his treatment of a case was in contemplation, it was unfortunate that he was not allowed an opportunity of being present at that postmortem examination in order that he might see for himself what was shown to elucidate the case. He was not there. The microscopical examination of the membrane might have assisted him for aught one knows. It is an unfortunate incident. I do not advise you to attach too much importance to it, but I do not think it right to pass it over without expressing my agreement with Sir. E. Marshall-Hall's statement.

Verdict
The jury deliberated for twenty minutes. On their return the foreman announced that they had agreed on a verdict of 'Not Guilty', an announcement which was received with loud applause in the crowded court. Dr Hadwen was accordingly discharged.

His mantra had always been 'Hold on and win.'

Comment: The judge's summing up was an excellent presentation to the jury to guide them as to how to come to a conclusion. In retrospect, clinical observation of diphtheria was debated, and also the reliability of interpreting throat swab culture. The usefulness and dangers of administering anti-toxin were brought into the evidence.

Once Dr Ellis took over treatment of Nellie, no communication was made by him to Hadwen as to the outcome and Hadwen received no notification of the postmortem examination.

Later, in the trial itself, it was revealed that there was a background of antagonism between Dr Ellis and Hadwen, indeed Dr Ellis had communicated by letter ahead of the trial objecting that his name might be associated with inaccurate certifying of cases of smallpox. Letters show Hadwen attempted a reconciliation. The next revelation was Hadwen had always been hounded for his views and attempts made to undermine his campaigning. During the time of Hadwen's trial in 1924, a patient of a Cheltenham doctor was informed by him that a fellow practitioner in the town had carried out a vaccination on Hadwen. The latter practitioner had since died so the accusation could not be challenged. This event could have had serious repercussions for Hadwen when his views were questioned in court. There followed a direct denial by Hadwen and this resulted in a public apology in print:-

> An Apology to Walter Hadwen, M. D. L. R. C. P., M. R. C. S., L. S. A. of Brunswick House, Gloucester.
> I————-M. D., C. M. of————Cheltenham, hereby admit that I did on the 29th day of October 1924, at Cheltenham, state that during the 1896 smallpox epidemic you were vaccinated by a Cheltenham doctor, which statement I now find to be without foundation, I hereby unreservedly withdraw the allegation, and express regret at having made the same. I have agreed to pay your solicitor costs and the cost of the publication of this apology. Dated 30th December, 1924.

The name of the offender has been removed. The date quoted does not really fit with the fact that Hadwen's trial was well finished at this time. Also, the evidence was that Hadwen had never even visited Cheltenham. The accounts of this event were made known in Canada when there were the reports of a second 'smallpox' outbreak in Gloucester in 1923.

The importance of the judgement was that a doctor was entitled to treat a patient entirely according to his own opinion and it was up to the patients to choose a doctor with a sound opinion. Hadwen aged 70yrs at the time. was correctly acquitted, the cause of death in doubt and antitoxin treatment was unlikely to have saved the child even if she had diphtheria.

Hadwen was quoted as saying: 'My success in life has depended entirely upon following my own counsels, and never paying the slightest attention to what anybody said if their views went contrary to my own'.

The court had been crowded each day of the trial and many people crowded the streets outside awaiting the verdict in the pouring rain. It is said their number was 5,000. Once released Hadwen was whisked away in his solicitor's car so quickly that he was unable to meet up with his wife and other family members. There are two versions of the immediate aftermath. Kidd reports that the solicitor's car then drove Hadwen towards his home and then diverted to Albion Hall where a crowd awaited. The Hall was packed where Hadwen addressed them for 20 minutes including an expression of sympathy towards the mother who had lost her child.

It was revealed that a fund had been raised by the workers in Gloucester to help defray the trial costs. This was augmented by his admirers who recognised his devotion to the anti-vivisection cause and

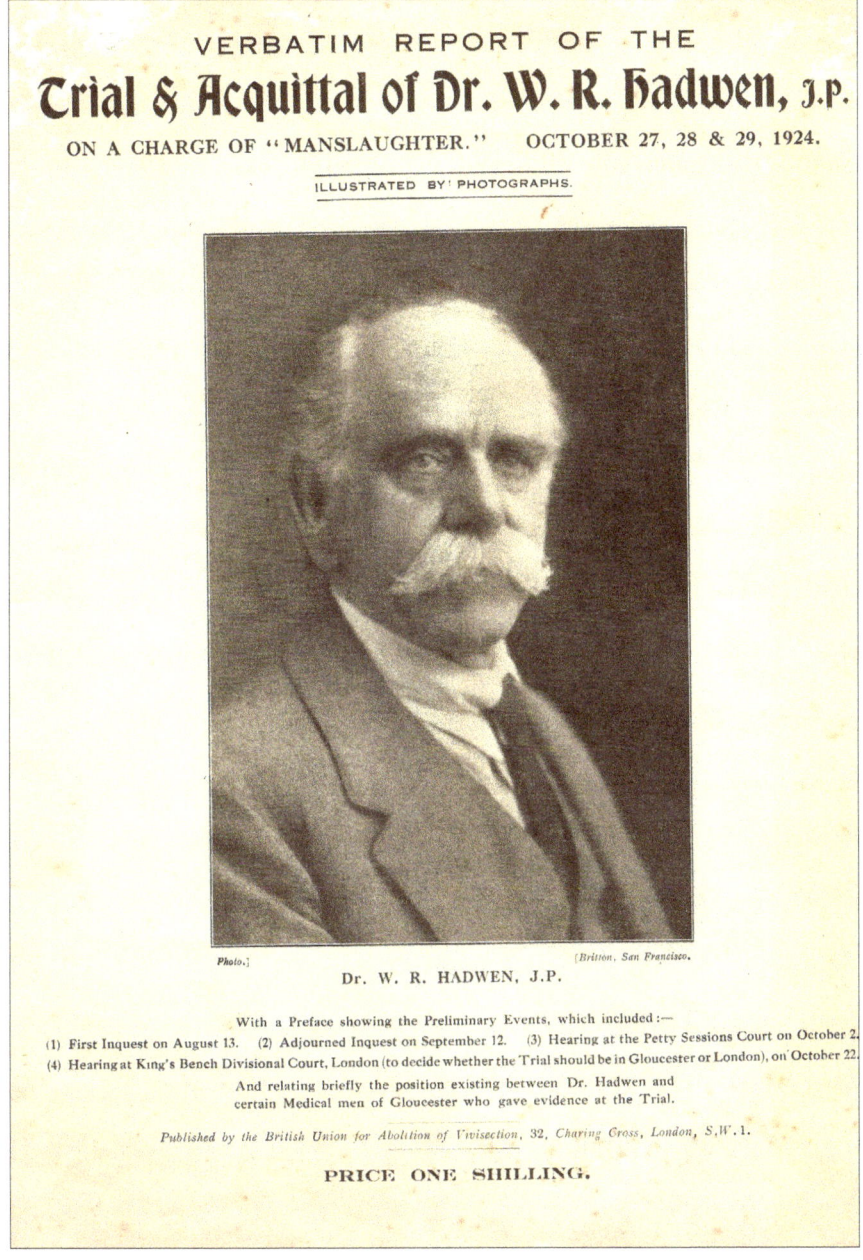

the total was sufficient to cover trial costs, as well as a great meeting in Queen's Hall, London at a later date, and it even covered the cost of printing the copies of the trial verbatim report.

Hadwen's granddaughter confirms that his supporters organised a thanksgiving meeting in Shire Hall which was packed and hundreds left outside. One version of events reports that the crowd welcomed him and carried him shoulder high into the building. The rector of St. Mary de Crypt spoke saying 'I formed the estimate of Dr Hadwen's character the first day I met him, each succeeding time of renewing his acquaintance has added to my first conviction that in him we have a remarkable honesty of purpose to act in any circumstances according to what he believes to be true and right, one with a heart which beats with active love for all humanity, man, woman, and child . . . ' Hadwen's wife was present to hear the tributes.

Afterwards a landau was waiting to carry Hadwen and family back to his home but the journey was accompanied by men carrying torches and a band playing marches.

He later spoke to members of the BUAV arranged at Caxton Hall in London saying he felt positive about the outcome and that things would come right.

The Queen's Hall was full for Hadwen's welcome and four doctors testified to having the same opinions as Hadwen. Congratulations were read from G. K. Chesterton, Bernard Shaw, John Galsworthy (who campaigned for animal welfare) and Miss Margaret Bondfield (Labour politician).

After resting a while, he took up his practice commitments again but not surprisingly the initial blow of his son's death and later his own public trial had worn him down.

On reflection, the circumstances of the trial hardly compare with the medico-legal support a doctor of today can experience. The Medical Defence Union was founded in 1885 but nowhere is there any hint that Hadwen took advice directly from such a body, and he was not a member of the BMA from which he could have sought assistance. In any case, he was so independent that he may well have rejected any advice from such organisations if it meant appeasement at any stage when facing the manslaughter charge.

11
CHILLINGHAM AND EARL OF TANKERVILLE

GEORGE MONTAGU BENNET (1852–1931) became the 7th Earl of Tankerville. He inherited his title in 1899. Apparently he was a bit of an adventurer and lived a colourful life. He was a midshipman, then a lieutenant in the Rifle Brigade. He went off to America and there for a time was a circus clown. He met his wife to be in New York and married her in Washington. She had been a music teacher and he became friends with the two evangelists and revivalists Sankey and Moody. He was known as 'The Singing Earl', singing hymns during his revival work both in America and UK. He had been trained as a professional singer. I can only deduce that his connection with Hadwen had blossomed, not only because of the Earl's conviction and support for the anti-vivisection movement via BUAV but also because of his Christian evangelical background.

The Earl had made his maiden speech in the House of Lords on the cause of anti-vaccination. He had chaired several meetings where Hadwen had been the main speaker. He and Hadwen and the Countess of Tankerville enjoyed each other's company.

After Hadwen's experiences of his trial he was delighted to receive an invitation to visit the Earl's estate at Chillingham Castle, near Alnwick, Northumberland. Originally a monastery, the castle was built around the 13th century. The Countess acted as guide, Hadwen was immediately captivated by the surroundings and his hostess gave him full detail of the family history and the castle's past. He was shown the dungeons and torture chamber and told the stories of the ghosts who were said to appear in the Castle.

One photograph exists, in documents handed to me, showing the Earl and Countess. Hadwen was accompanied by his elder daughter, Una, her husband and their daughter. Again Hadwen's wife seems not

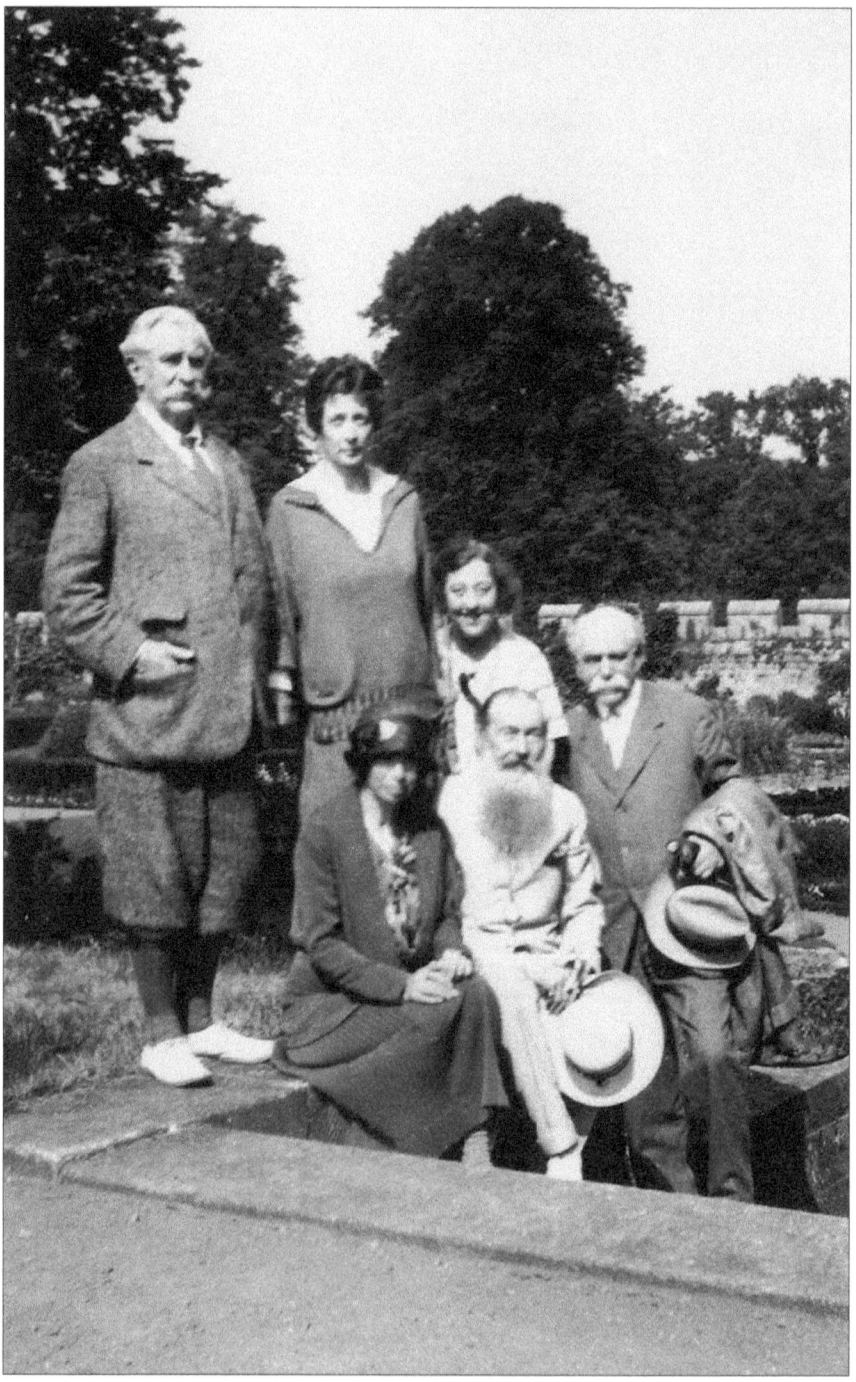

The Earl, Countess, Hadwen's granddaughter, and in front, Una with husband and Hadwen.

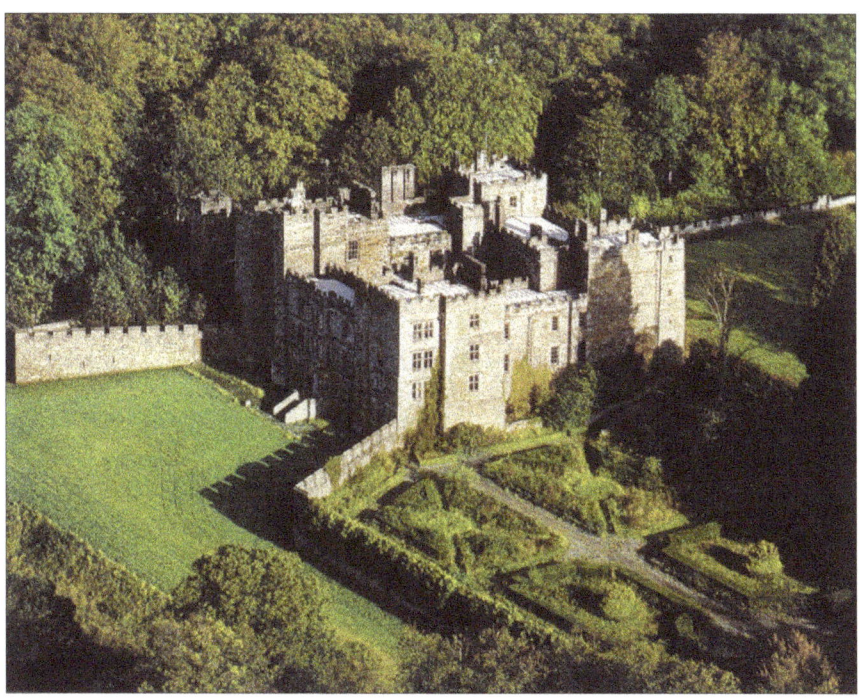

Modern images of the castle and grounds. The steps up to the castle where the photograph of Hadwen's visit was taken and be clearly seen

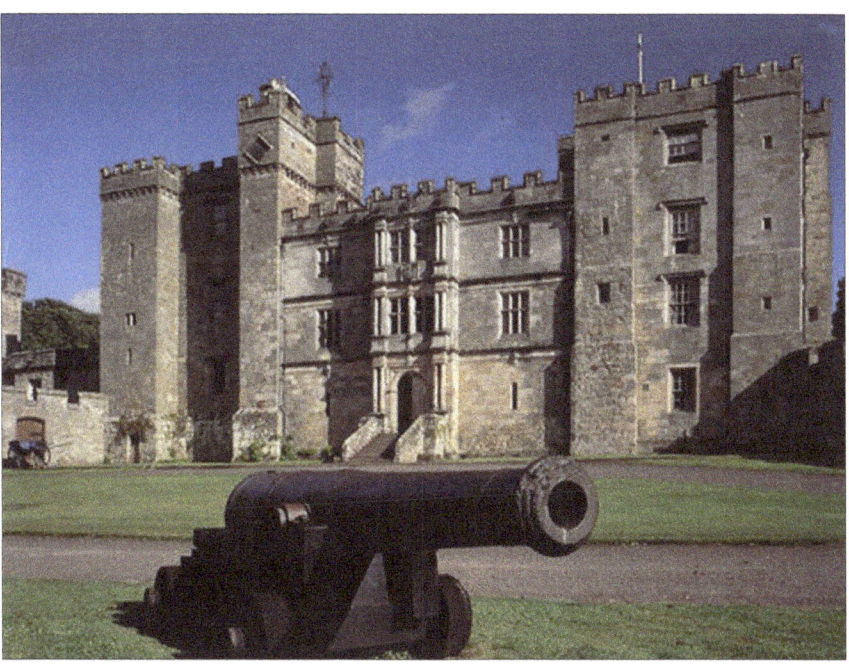

to feature. This was a visit for a short time, probably a day or two. The rest of his family members, totalling four in number, possibly only met there for the day as they lived in the North-East. Hadwen stayed over at least one night as he describes the bedroom in which he slept. Una, living in the area, no doubt was able to join Hadwen as a family outing to meet up at Chillingham. This was in July 1925.

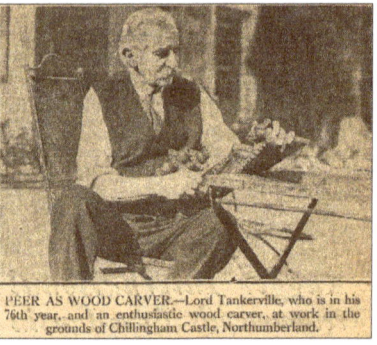

A cutting from 1928 newspaper article which shows the Earl at his workbench following his hobby of wood carving

Taking the facts as I understand the situation, it seems quite remarkable that Hadwen sat down, once home, and produced a complete description of the castle room by room. The original document I have is typed, not handwritten, and takes up 20 pages.

It starts 'Eight miles from Belford station, along country lanes, over extensive moors, through scattered villages and past an occasional farm, we reach the ancestral home of the Tankervilles, hidden behind a high unbroken wall nine miles in circumference which encircles the park and Castle of Chillingham'. The script is a complete guide for a visitor and includes the family history and detail of all the paintings

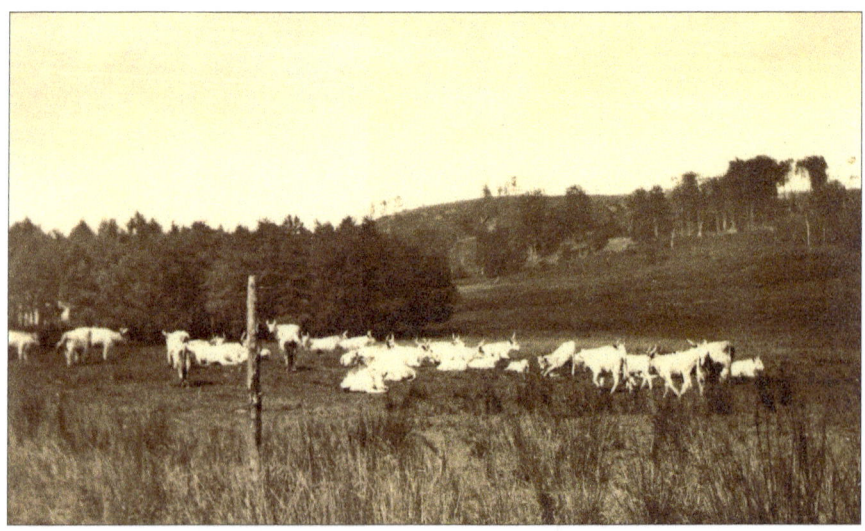

Old image (? by Hadwen) from the 1900's showing the herd at Chillingham Park.

mounted on the walls of the dining hall. Hadwen describes the Earl's talent for woodcarving and earlier in his life, his painting talent. Not long before Hadwen's visit the Earl opened the castle grounds to some 2,000 guests and the 70 year old Earl entertained them by singing in the great courtyard.

After the death of the Earl, apparently many of the contents were disposed of and the castle became poorly maintained. It is now owned by Sir Humphry Wakefield Bt. and is being gradually restored.

The next item Hadwen refers to is 'The Wild Cattle of Chillingham' who exist and remain free and wild but enclosed in Chillingham Park for the last 700 years. There is no human interference or management of a breeding programme. The herd numbers vary but 100 beasts is the average who roam the 1,000 acre protected park. They have been genetically isolated for hundreds of years. In case of disease eg. foot and mouth disease, there is a small reserve of around 20 animals on a Crown Estate in Scotland. Inbreeding does not seem to have weakened the herd. Again, amongst material handed to me is a photograph of the cattle at the time and probably taken by Hadwen with his Kodak, and I have no doubt that Hadwen was very respectful of the preservation of this herd without any animal cruelty or veterinary interference. They are endangered and, as a breed, rarer than panda or mountain gorilla. Everything as nature had intended. Alongside the herd, the park area provides a safe haven for European green woodpecker, nuthatch and red squirrel, and also roe and fallow deer. The herd is now protected by a Trust. Further reference to Chillingham will be made later.

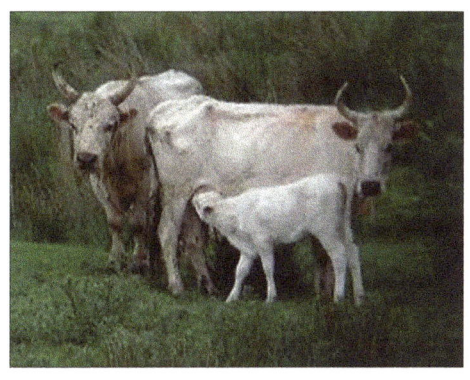

"The White Cattle" today with calf suckling, horns have black tips and brown hair within their ears.

12
THE TRAVELLER

Recording in chronological order the considerable travels that Hadwen undertook is not without difficulty.

In the Bibliography I have indicated only some of the talks and lectures he gave in various venues in UK to show his travels.

I have already mentioned his holiday in 1884 which included visiting Brussels, Luxembourg, Basle, Berne and Lucerne. This was followed by a short visit to Paris with his wife in 1891.

He crossed to the Isle of Man in 1913 to give evidence to the Legislative Council to support conscientious objectors to vaccination. This venture was followed in 1914 when he completed his journey to Malta aboard the *S.S. Simla* of the Peninsular and Oriental Steam Navigation Company. The main purpose was to investigate Brucellosis (Undulent or Malta Fever). The controversy was as to whether this 'disease' was as a result of overcrowding and poor sanitation or due to the newly discovered germ. The latter had been researched by a Maltese pathologist and then by Col. Bruce who, at first, did not feel the original research proved the source of the problem but eventually approved the conclusions and took the credit. Goat's milk was said to be the source of the problem and Hadwen's statistics showed that inaccuracies had occurred in presenting the facts to the Royal Commission. He was most concerned that goats were being unnecessarily slaughtered and he also proved that when the Army personnel were billeted in new accommodation with modern facilities Malta Fever was no longer a risk, whereas when the Navy remained stationed at the harbour in poor conditions the fever persisted. He reported back to BUAV with his findings and it may be they funded his expenses.

It is mentioned that Hadwen did employ locum tenens for his longer absences from the Practice. How he managed to cover the cost for many of his meetings he undertook remains a mystery and how the patients reacted to his non-availability is not mentioned.

In his book *First Impressions of America* he describes visiting Venice in Los Angeles he compares it with an earlier visit to Venice and Florence though I have not been able to confirm this trip.

In 1905 Hadwen was under a lot of pressure to take over as an officer in the BUAV and in particular I have mentioned he had to use some of his own monies to cover the organisation's expenses. However, one day he received a letter enclosed in a cigar box, which at first sight he thought a hoax, but it was worded as follows:

Dear Sir, Four admirers of your work in the Anti-vivisection Cause who are aware that you do not spare yourself, and who fear that your health will give way if you do not take more rest, are anxious that you should, at the earliest date possible, take a complete holiday. Knowing that you have to consider the responsibilities of a family and the claims of the causes in which you are interested, they hope that you will not object to their defraying the cost of such holiday, which they consider a privilege, and they send herewith the sum of £100, trusting that you will consider yourself bound by honour to spend it in the way indicated.

The time of the holiday you will, of course, choose according to your own convenience and the necessities of your practice, but they beg to express the hope that you will not delay many months, lest a collapse in health should come upon you which might have been avoided if you had taken the matter in time. The four friends who beg your acceptance of this gift are actuated as much by a desire for the welfare of the Anti-vivisection Cause, which so largely depends on you, as by personal regard and warm gratitude for the services you have rendered it.'

In token that you have received the money they would be much obliged if you would insert in the 'Agony column' of the *Standard* for Saturday, February 25th, or, failing that, the following Monday or Tuesday, this announcement,

'Received-one hundred. Agree to terms. Walter R.

The biographer, Kidd, understandably withheld the names of the donors.

Hadwen's reaction was to exclaim that at last he would see Palestine. On travelling to Alexandria he met, by chance, a fellow doctor and anti-vaccinationist who took it upon himself to show Hadwen all the sights. Next came Cairo and then on to Palestine. There he journeyed by horseback or mule. He was able to view many of the biblical sites and made notes which were used for articles in the local *Citizen* newspaper. On his return journey he made time to include viewing the ruins of Karnak and Luxor.

There is an incidental story of Hadwen visiting Rome and it may well be that it was on this visit that he included Venice and Florence. Again the sequence of these sightseeing events is uncertain but this tour must have been before the First World War. Rome included the Vatican but he was told that it was impossible for him to gain entry. However a stranger invited him to join his family in the Audience Chamber, but it was stipulated that they were to conform to the rules of etiquette and to kneel in line. If the Pope extended his hand, he should put his lips to the 'Apostolic Ring' on his finger. Hadwen, having agreed to the protocol, forthwith forgot the instruction. He only bowed registering the size and carving of the ring and kissed the Pope's hand instead. Apparently this caused offence at the Vatican and rules were tightened about admitting Protestants!

The year 1921 saw Hadwen make his prolonged visit to America. This adventure is all recorded in his book *First Impressions of America*, which I have summarised in an Appendix to this book. He needed rest and it was thought that sightseeing in America would revitalise him. True to form he was writing to record every part of the journey, but he did seem to be refreshed and stated he had never felt so fit. He enjoyed American hospitality mainly supplied by the anti-vivisectionist groups in every area visited. It was all quite an undertaking for a 67-year-old. His first experience of everyone expecting a tip which he found inexplicable and expensive! Wherever he went his addresses to very formal meetings and dinners were lauded and congratulations were heaped upon him. His return journey on this tour is not specified in his own book but Kidd says he returned on the Cunard liner *Aquitania* apparently from New York in July 1921. My search to find his outward journey and identify his cabin number is mentioned in the Summary. However, some sixteen months after he got back to Gloucester he was invited to return to the USA. A referendum on vivisection was to be taken in California and Hadwen was requested to 'come over and help'. Again his movements were recorded in the *Abolitionist* magazine during 1923. Passenger lists show him departing from Southampton to New York on 13 September, 1922 sailing on the '*Olympic*' of the White Star line. In Montreal he was unexpectedly abused and even accused of being a liar. He responded with courtesy and calmness. In Toronto he was accused to his face of being a rascal. Another letter in a local paper accused him of being a paid agitator. He moved on to Chicago where the editor of the *Journal of the American Medical Association* put pen to paper by making an abusive personal attack. Moving on he visited and spoke in Minneapolis, Spokane and Seattle. On his way to this last city the train broke down in the mountains and was delayed for more than two hours. He took the opportunity to walk out into the forest and visited a family in a log cabin offering payment for a cup of tea. In talking to the housewife, she told him her son had been in the War and had been inoculated and vaccinated which had caused him to spend five months in hospital and thereafter his life was ruined. She went on to say that she had read in a Sunday paper that a doctor who had come from England had stated that many poor fellows had been killed by it and that it didn't do any good anyhow. Hadwen declared he was that doctor and the lady was astonished and refused any payment for the tea.

After Seattle and also visiting Vancouver he took a sea voyage for two days to San Francisco. The local paper headed an article on 'Medical Research and Vivisection' by a Professor of Research Medicine which contained the following comment most certainly directed against Hadwen's arrival.

> Unfortunately there are a few aged individuals with medical degrees who are willing to earn their living by vilifying the great leaders of their profession, and attempting to prove that medicine has not moved in the slightest since 1850. No educated person today can be taken in by such arguments.

Typically, Hadwen replied that he could be justified in earning a living by lecturing in defence of animals more than the professor by torturing them. He followed by stressing he sacrificed income to defend animal cruelty nor ever accepted a fee for any lecture he gave. This all brought much publicity to his advantage. He claimed, however, that he had been subjected to insults and abuse by members of his profession in USA which would have been impossible on a British platform. Whatever, he later succeeded in attaining his interview with President Harding whose views were straightforward, open and sincere which Hadwen suggested were the makings of a great man.

Passenger lists show his return to Southampton from New York on the *Majestic* of the White Star Line. This tour took some eleven weeks.

The official record of Hadwen's trial also shows that, to help him recuperate, his friend, a fellow J.P., invited Hadwen to join him in a short tour of Devon and Cornwall. This must have been a relaxing experience by being chauffeur driven in a semi-convertible Rolls-Royce!

By the age of 72 years, Hadwen's life had, to say the least, been turbulent with the death of his son and then his trial for manslaughter. He had travelled extensively through America and expressed some reluctance to return the second time in 1923 as such trips involved many public speaking engagements. It seemed he was becoming weary and tiring of constant debate and argument for his cause. He no longer sought any form of adulation, preferring time to reflect away from constant company.

However, he decided in 1926 that there was more of the world he wished to explore and so he set off to join the *Franconia* Cunard liner at Monaco. No family members accompanied him but once more, he wrote a travel record to be sent back to the Gloucester *Citizen* newspaper for everyone to follow his experiences. The voyage appears to have refreshed him. His ports of call included Egypt, India and Taj Mahal, Ceylon, Dutch East Indies, Singapore, the Philippines and China. He was probably abroad for some eight weeks or more. Passenger records show he travelled on a return journey on the *Franconia* from Yokohama to New York in May 1926 and after two weeks boarded the *Franconia* again to travel to Liverpool via Boston. He seemed to admire all the advantage the Empire was giving to our dominions and colonies. This view was expressed, once he returned to Britain, and was addressing a Rotary Club with illustrations by lantern slides. This talk was to the Gloucester Rotary Club, the only Rotary Club in the city at that time. The Club has a complete archive of their meetings since their formation in 1920 and they confirm the talk on Friday, 6 July 1926 entitled 'Impressions of World Tour' with 65 members present and four guests at the Spread Eagle Hotel. He told the story of how, on arriving in Honolulu, Hawaii, passengers were to prove they are vaccinated within the last 12 months. The penalty was quarantine in Honolulu. Hadwen was supported by three other anti-vaccinators as he challenged the rule. It was then announced that a mark, however discernible, on the arm, would suffice as evidence of protection and 'red tape' was satisfied.

So concluded his voyages abroad and his travels around England became less frequent.

13
HADWEN'S LAST YEARS AND DEATH

AT THE AGE of 72 years and after his world cruise, Hadwen settled back into routine family practice in Gloucester. Evenings were probably spent in more correspondence. In April 1928 He was able to celebrate his Golden Wedding Anniversary. It was suggested to him that he might take on an assistant, but financial constraints in the economic depression made him cautious about additional expenditure.

Within the BUAV, which he had nurtured over many years, his control and ideas were beginning to be challenged, if covertly. An important meeting, the annual Council meeting of BUAV was held in June 1932; he knew there were rumblings of some discontent and he actually was heckled. He continued as elected President but his energies were failing and he admitted that controversy of any kind was a great strain. Physically he was becoming breathless and he recognised that his heart was weakening. Hadwen managed to attend his next but last committee meeting in the October and went on to have tea with his daughter who lived in Golders Green. She reported he looked tired but the Council meeting had gone better than expected, however, he commented, there was a lot still to be achieved but time was short for him now. Hadwen's final committee meeting of the BUAV on 10 November, 1932 was a more relaxed affair with plenty of goodwill from his fellow members. He was able to negotiate the tube in Trafalgar Square to get to Paddington Station. At this point he confessed to his secretary, who had made sure he got on to his train, that he might only last a month or two more and at that, the train departed to Gloucester and Kidd, his secretary and biographer, never saw him again. He had developed a trembling hand and had difficulty holding a pen.

He wrote to his friend that he had 'collapsed' on his way walking to Albion Hall, a short distance from Brunswick Square, to hear a choir practice. Apparently he eventually arrived but was greatly troubled by breathlessness. He wrote to a friend 'I am done for!' and also reported that diabetes had been diagnosed. He cancelled a planned meeting he was to attend in Nottingham on 8 December. Soon after this episode a further collapse occured on his way to attend a Bible Class and a car had to be found to take him home. This resulted in him finally 'taking to his bed'.

It is described that he sent for his friend, Dr Alcock, to thoroughly examine his heart. This physician's name has not been mentioned at any point until now and it is not clear whether he was a Consultant Physician or General Practitioner. No treatment was offered as it was said his heart muscle was irretrievably damaged.

All engagements were cancelled and letters dictated. A locum was engaged who Hadwen had thought might become an assistant and take over his practice as his views were compatible with Hadwen's beliefs. His daughter, Una Rodenhurst travelled from London to comfort him. Being the fighter he was he recovered enough to be taken out for one or two drives into the countryside. On Christmas Day, the family congregated around his bed and listened to some stories of his travels.

As the reader might expect, despite his worsening condition Hadwen had dictated his sermon and arrangements for the Christmas Day evening service. This too has survived in full text of four typed pages and includes hymn choices and carols by the choir. He stated the tunes to be used for the hymns which used specified Sankey tunes for two carols. This choice may have been influenced by his friend the Earl of Tankerville's association with Sankey and Moody. The title of the sermon was 'The Incarnation' . He writes that the scriptures were inspired by the Holy Spirit and can give individuals a clear message. The New Testament is the fulfilment of the old. He defines Christ as King and Messiah, Prophet and teacher, Son of Man and finally Word of God. The content continues to take a very basic theme with much quoting from Bible passages. Some would criticise that it was more of a lecture than an inspiration. But Hadwen's Christian belief never faltered until his dying day.

As he lay in his bed, even at the last, he was dictating letters. Finally there was a crash in the bedroom, instantly Hadwen's wife and daughter were there and found him having fallen across a bedside table which had broken. He told his daughter he thought he was dying. Dr Alcock arrived and was able to lift him back into his bed hardly conscious. The Doctor was only able to offer comfort rather than medication and

Hadwen very shortly died peacefully on 27 December 1932. A report stated that he died of 'cardiac asthma' (heart failure).

Announcements were made in all the principle newspapers in UK and the news cabled to Canada and USA.

On 31 December 1932 the funeral service was held in a crowded Albion Hall (in those days it could hold 500 people). The service was conducted by Mr Russell Elliott a barrister-at-law. We have no detail of who this person was as his name has not been mentioned before. Hadwen was buried near the little chapel in what is now the 'Old Cemetery" in Gloucester. The coffin was carried by the brethren of Albion Hall. There were many people gathered there but also many patients waited outside the surgery in Barton Street to witness the funeral; but to their disappointment the procession went in a more direct route at the request of the police, because the expected crowds might cause traffic congestion. Mourners included the Mayor and representatives of the city Corporation and Magistrate's Bench.

The *Abolitionist* published a special memorial edition in the February 1933 issue, the author being Beatrice Kidd.

Hadwen's wife died some eight months later and she was buried alongside her husband. The site of the grave was chosen with assistance of the Cemetery caretaker who mentioned that Hadwen had often stood

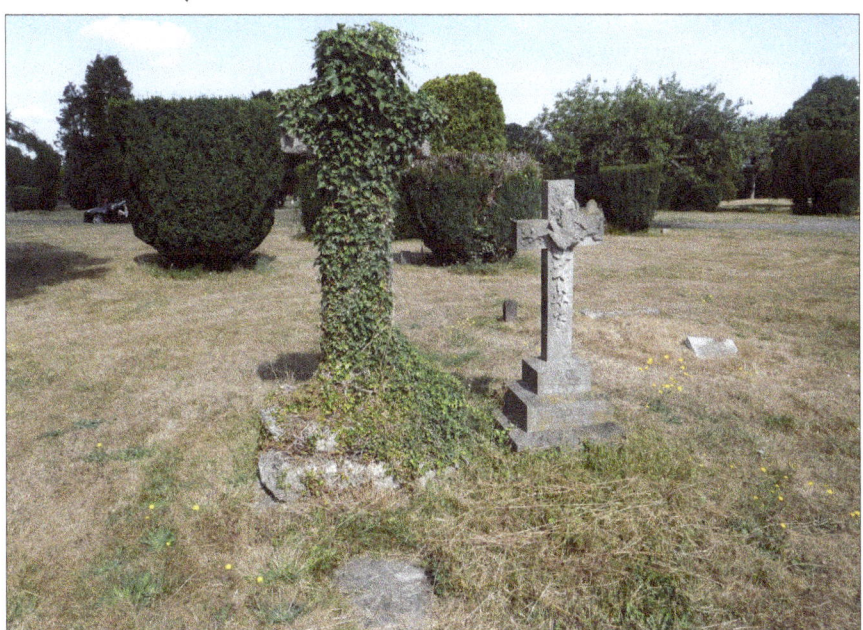

The overgrown grave in Gloucester old cemetery

on this favoured spot alongside the Cemetery Chapel when attending patient's and friend's interments.

At first there was a simple family tombstone to mark the spot. But the BUAV and other admirers set about raising a Memorial Fund and by 1935 nearly £700 was donated. The memorial was designed by an architect and a cross erected of undressed rugged Cotswold stone at the head of the grave. Originally a tablet of commemoration was included, made by a local stonemason, with a surrounding stone border outlining the grave itself. Though not in total disrepair, the cross stands but the border stones have been removed. The dedication, которая is now barely discernible, read :-

> Walter Robert Hadwen, JP., MD
> President of the Union for the Abolition of Vivisection
> 3rd August, 1854
> 27th December, 1932.
> and
> Alice Caroline Mackenzie Hadwen
> 26th April, 1850
> 11th August, 1933.
>
> Teach us, Good Lord,
> To serve thee as Thou deservest,
> To give and not to count the cost,
> To fight and not to heed the wounds,
> To toil and not to seek for rest,
> To labour and not to ask for any reward,
> Save that of knowing that we do Thy will.

Until the Memorial was completed, the grave was tended twice a week and flowers left to enhance the grave itself. The granddaughter obtained permission to plant an ivy at the base of the cross and areas were fashioned for flowering plants. Also, a 'bowl' was designed to contain bird seed or bread. Even at this point, controversy was not far away and complaints made to the Town Clerk that birds arrived in great numbers and their droppings caused a nuisance. An official letter was sent to ask friends and family to desist from this action.

The *Abolitionist*, in January 1935, gave a full description of the 'Hadwen Memorial' which was opened by Mrs Leo (Una) Rodenhurst,

Hadwen's daughter. This was the frontage of the BUAV office at 47, Whitehall. This was now a permanent shop, fitted with a non-reflecting glass window and handsome facade, making a most imposing and up-to-date advertisement for anti-vivisection. The frontage was matched with a beautiful lecture and meeting room behind and storage space for literature. All this designed for the continuing work of BUAV and recognised as the best known propaganda centre for the Movement. The interior had been tastefully decorated and included light oak panelling which gave a dignified atmosphere. A long lease for the property had been negotiated.

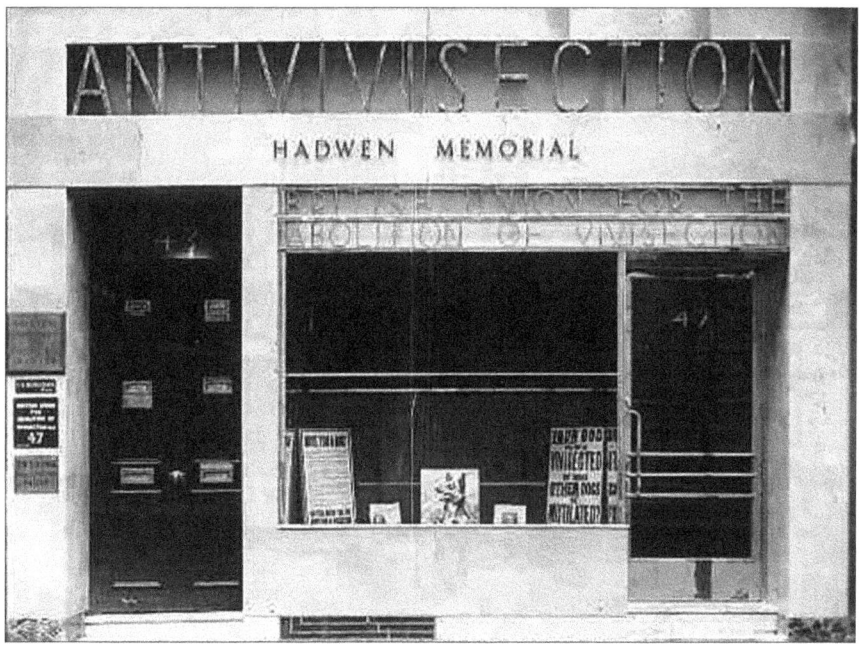

The Hadwen Memorial Window, 47 Whitehall, London containing the anti-vivisection shop

The opening ceremony took place on 10 December, 1934. The President of BUAV at that time was Leonora Countess of Tankerville. She, along with Viscount and Viscountess Harberton and supporting Parliamentary Members regretfully had to offer apologies for non-attendance due to a vote in Parliament. Apparently Countess Tankerville had had a recent accident. Towards the end of the tribute, those attending the opening experienced listening to Hadwen's voice from the recording mentioned in Chapter 7. (There is no further specific clue as to an exact date of the recording but it was said he made the recording 'several years ago'),

The *Citizen* published Hadwen's will on 24 February 1933 reporting that he left £14, 862 and, as has been already stated, left a bequest of £2, 500 for Gertrude Best recognising her devotion to the Albion Hall Choir and Music. There was also recognition to children and grandchildren, servants and his wife who had security of the house for her life.

Much later, in August 1954, a memorial service to Hadwen was held at his graveside to mark the centenary of his birth. More than 50 people attended including Grace Newman, Hadwen's daughter. There were floral tributes from the Gloucester branch of the BUAV, and BUAV headquarters and many other branches, some representatives of these branches being present in person. Specifically mentioned was a member of the Nelson Street Mission. Tributes were expressed, 'In proud and grateful memory', 'in loving remembrance', 'in memory of a great and good man', 'in remembrance of a great and fearless man'. Prayers and an address were given by a Rev. Keith Pilcher, vicar of Alveston, in which he mentioned Hadwen's indifference to public opinion, his complete confidence in himself, supreme optimism and trust in God. Quoted was his motto 'hold on and win'.

Subsequent developments after Hadwen's death need to be recorded rather than it being assumed that his name and life have been forgotten.

14
'THERAPEUTICS'

I HAVE TRIED to follow Hadwen's first career in Pharmacy and more detail of the types of medication used in his time and is worthwhile recording to give some idea of products and prescribing at the time of Hadwen's training and practice.

The following prescription was forwarded to me by a chemist in Highbridge who found the detail in an old internal recipe note book found in 'Orchard's Chemists', Highbridge.

'Hadwen's Chlorodyne'

Opium Tincture 2 fl. oz.
Sulphuric Ether 1. 5 fl. oz
Water half fl. oz
Chloroform 2 fl. oz
Burnt Sugar Solution 2 fl. oz
Dilute Hydrocyanic Acid half fl. oz
Capsicum Tincture 180 minims
Peppermint Essence 180 minims

This is a typical Victorian recipe for a cough !

There is mentioned in *Hadwen of Gloucester* that when Hadwen was not feeling well with pain and loss of energy he took pills made up of 'Dandelion, Chamomile, Quinine and Rhubarb' which made him a new man! When, again feeling unwell, a visiting friend insisted he take oatmeal porridge with brandy in it, intruding on his teetotal principles! In a letter, he gives his father a list of drugs he also took when feeling unwell:-

Calomel: mercury chloride/purgative! odourless/poisonous
Croton Oil: from a tree cultivated in India, foul smelling, potent purgative
Black Draught: Commercial liquid syrup laxative. Senna and magnesia

One assumes he did not take doses of these products all together!

On a later occasion, Hadwen mentions, when a GP, giving Vinegar in hot water as a gargle to a child with a throat infection and in addition painting the throat with glycerine. A tonic prescribed was 'Syrup of phosphiate Mixture' (this might have been misspelt)

IN PREVIOUS CHAPTERS I have tried to tell the story of Hadwen's life as accurately as I can and to include much of the additional information I have collected since the original biography in 1932. Up till this chapter I have kept as strictly as possible to historic facts but now begin to record subsequent events which had a personal association.

As my interest in the general history of the practice grew and I heard the patient's stories and memories I began to slowly gather memorabilia which, in the end, produced an unexpected 'side effect'.

The practice had abandoned the old surgery in Barton Street in the early 1970s but I was able to obtain permission to explore the old chemist shop, 'Duckworths', which has remained disused since. The old surgery premises has been divided into apartments for private rental. As this happened, our more central and modernised building at 25a Park Road became the main surgery which was gradually further modernised and extended to meet demand.

Once access had been achieved, the basement was found to be full of rubble but some old bottles had survived. I was able to remove a few undamaged examples , known as 'stock bottles' without labels. Cleaned up, as a group, they were colourful and displayed well. At almost the same time my wife and I visited a village show and there was a stall of old bottles for sale. The vendor was happy to enthuse my interest in the medicines and eventually Quack Cures. A hobby of collecting had started.

Examples of labels of stock products used in the pharmacies in Hadwen's day are illustrated on page 31, which give a little insight into prescribing habits.

Next, I became aware of John Wesley's book, aptly named *Primitive Physic*, first published in 1747. My copy is dated 1761 and on these pages shows two famous medicines and how to make them. The idea

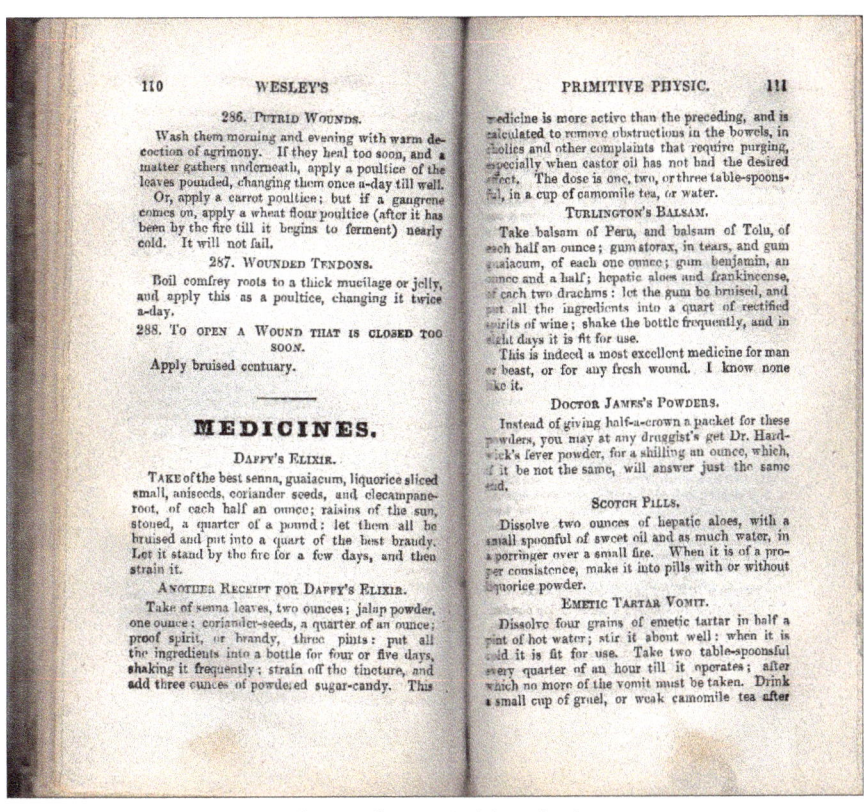

John Wesley's Primitive Physic

was to bring practical medical advice to workers who could not afford private doctors or the cost of medication. He gave good advice about healthy living, including fresh air and a balanced diet, also, as already mentioned, a cold shower each morning! The ailments with treatment are arranged in alphabetical order from 'Ague' to 'Wounds'.

The next point of interest was to discover two editions by the BMA entitled *Secret Remedies* in 1909 and *More Secret Remedies* in 1912. These manuals give detailed information about the manufacturer, their advertising techniques, prices, analysis and mark up price on the actual contents which was often considerable. Magical names were used. For example 'Dipsocure' and 'Antidipso' offering a permanent cure for the craving for alcohol! A box of two types of powders at 9 shillings was all that was needed to be effective. The contents were Acetanilide (6 parts) a toxic material for pain and raised temperature, Potassium Bromide (35 parts) which was used to calm and prevent fits. Add to these some sugar of milk (?lactose 59 parts) ingredients cost 1/3 of a penny. This gives

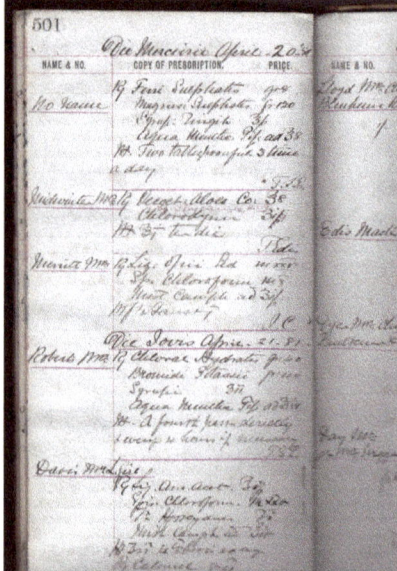 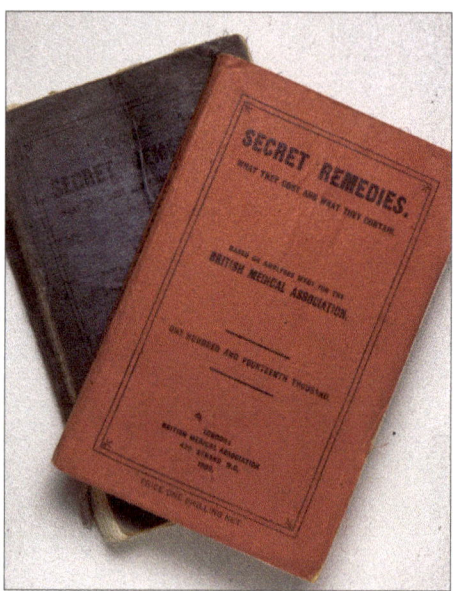

left: A prescribing day book rescued from another pharmacy. 1880 copper plate writing.
right: The Two BMA publications on 'Secret Remedies

the picture as to how clever marketing could make a fortune for the purveyor. There was no control over contents and classification for these commercial products available over the counter. These publications became an alert to the pharmacy and medical profession and eventually the Pure Food and Drugs Act came into law in America and then UK in the early 1900s. The claim to 'Cure' was dropped and became illegal but could be replaced by the wording 'Remedy' or 'Medicine' etc. All these commercial products were available over the counter or advised at consultation with a family doctor

In 1910 Hadwen embarked on correspondence by letter with the *BMJ* on a debate as to whether the Diphtheria anti-toxin benefitted mankind. In hindsight, he argues on evidence and statistic, that in the past Diphtheria was probably classified as 'Croup' and this altered the proof as to how effective the anti-toxin had been. Bacterial Diphtheria carriers were identified but had no clinical symptoms. Epidemics came in waves worldwide and therefore it was difficult for anyone to argue that any specific treatment was effective. He showed that figures recorded a fall in the number of deaths from diphtheria even before antitoxin was used and then an increase in the years after antitoxin therapy was introduced. The editor of the journal seems to have stopped further debate and left the judgement to the medical profession. After all, they had 15 years experience of using the antitoxin not only in this country but over all the civilised world!

The next set of correspondence in the *BMJ*, which involved Hadwen in 1910, was on the subject of the effectiveness of Capt. Feilden's Crimson Cross remedies and Ointment. Full details were published of the analysis and claims made. An advertisement appeared in the *Vaccination Enquirer* headed 'The Crimson Cross Remedies for fevers, measles, small-pox, influenza, pneumonia, pleurisy etc. renders the patient non-infectious'. Hadwen's name appeared in that advertisement as a source of statistics, though he denied any knowledge of this. The treatment was stated to be a simple solution to the vaccination problem. Hadwen did not claim it was a cure but was capable of ameliorating the pitting and scarring experienced in severe smallpox cases. Hadwen's belief in bathing and use of oils emphasised his faith in the remedy more for the property of the linseed oil contained therein than the other ingredients!

Content of the remedy was: Copper oleate; Anhydrous sodium sulphate; Beeswax; Resin (from pines and conifers); Linseed oil.

He describes its use in smallpox cases in Gloucester. His opposer was quite offensive in his letters in reply and Hadwen defended himself without rancour. There were written challenges in the *BMJ* as to the effectiveness of the remedies and this was linked with debate in writing on antivivisection. In one letter he describes how he was invited by the secretary of Charing Cross Medical Society to give a lecture and then a debate on the subject of Experiments on Living Animals, a storm broke out as a result of a petition by the vivisection party. The original Hon Sec. who had organised the lecture had been replaced and the newly appointed Secretary informed him the lecture had been cancelled. So much for freedom of speech! Hadwen stated that 'public speaking, however, forms my chief recreation from a busy practice'.

The analysis of the Crimson Cross remedies also showed the cost of the chemicals used and the retail price charged. The profit margin was more than substantial.

I then discovered that, not only was there concern about the claims and profits made by commercial medicine manufacturers but also mounting awareness of the risks and deaths from accidental poisoning when such liquids were ingested by mistake. There were some rules about clear labelling of bottles containing dangerous fluid but nothing else. The race was on to patent foolproof containers (glass or ceramic) for poisonous materials. 'Skull and Crossbones' was the visual sign for danger, as it still is. Ingenious designs were developed and patents registered. The 1908 Poisons and Pharmacy Act made it lawful only to place liquid poisons, if retailed to the public, in containers distinguishable by touch from ordinary bottles. The habit by the public of taking any old empty bottle to the apothecary and getting it filled up with some dangerous poisonous household product like bleach were gone! Many cases were recorded of accidental death by self poisoning when unlabelled substances were ingested. There was no point in putting such poisons into a bottle and using a gummed label that would come off. Colour, especially blue glass, was not an indicator necessarily of danger or caution. It became practice to have the word 'poison' or 'poisonous' or 'not to be taken' to be embossed on the glass. If you had poor eyesight or poor lighting or you were even illiterate, wording did not convey a danger. The solution was a container of distinctive shape to be easily identified by touch. Such designs have become a collector's passion.

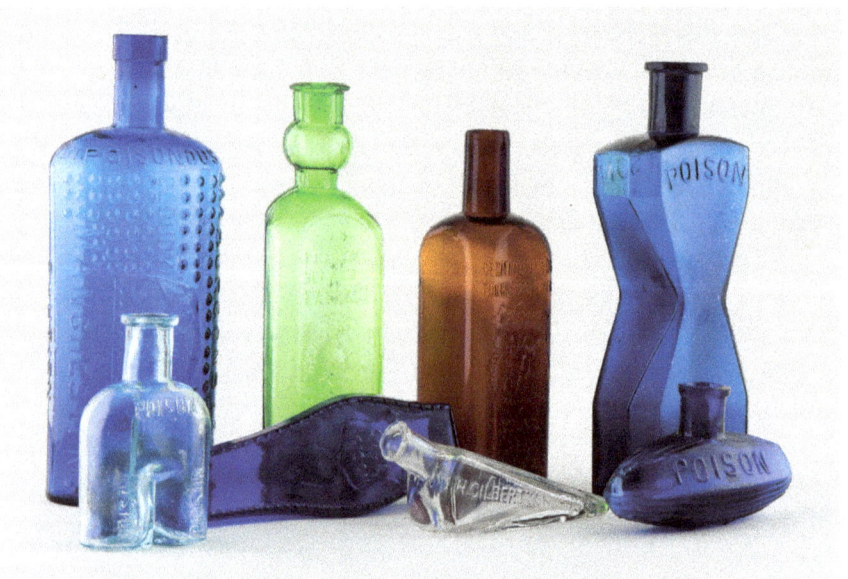

Burgons Ammonia(p) Fishers Manx Shrub(m) Radam's Microbe Killer(m) Wasp Waist(p)
Binocular(p) Coffin(p) Gilbertson's Wedge(p) Submarine(p)
p=poison   m= medicine

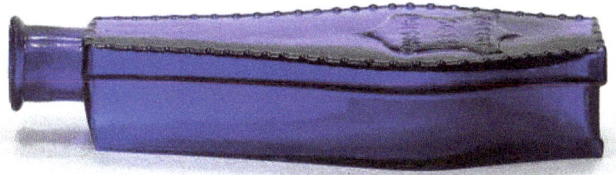

Detail of 'Coffin Poison' embossed 'Poison' with lid and nails! Only 6 examples have been recorded

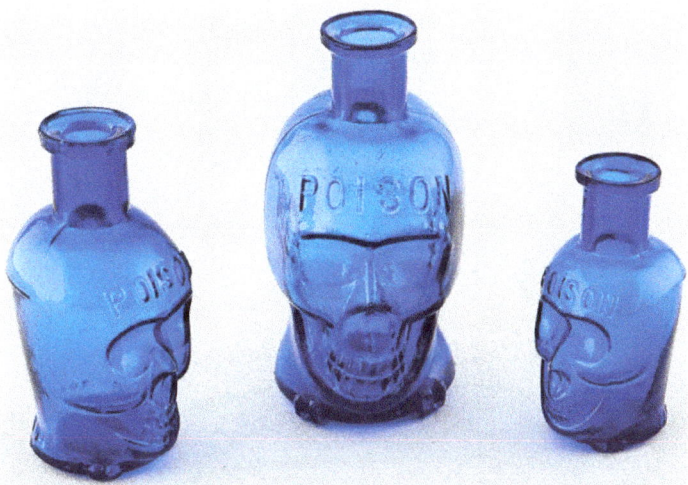

Rare full set of English 'Skull' poisons Patent 1894 with crossbones moulded on the base

LAMPLOUGH'S
PYRETIC SALINE.

HAVE IT IN YOUR HOUSES AND TRAVELS, USING NO OTHER; it gives instant relief in Headaches, Sea or Bilious Sickness, and quickly relieves or cures the worst form of Eruptive or Skin Complaints. The various diseases arising from Constipation, the Liver, or Blood Impurities, Inoculation, the results of breathing air infected with **Fevers, Measles, or Small-Pox**, are frequently prevented and certainly cured by its use.
 The great reputation of this remedy has called forth spurious imitations; beware of these fraudulent preparations—persons guilty of such conduct would for the purpose of gain rob the public of their health as soon as the proprietor of his well-earned fame and reward. Observe my name and trade mark as above, on a **buff-coloured wrapper**, without which the Saline cannot be genuine—113, Holborn Hill, London, E.C. Sold by all Chemists, and the Maker, in patent glass-stoppered bottles, at 2s. 6d., 4s. 6d, 11s. and 21s. each. [4

This product is the only one I found with a direct claim to cure smallpox. The bottle is relatively common with the name 'Lamplough's Pyretic Saline' embossed but the labelling in good condition is difficult to find.

As any collector will appreciate, seeking more examples of 'Quack Cures', both English and American became an obsession. It soon became clear that this is a worldwide hobby and rarities now claim a high price.

In the meantime, my wife, as a health visitor, became interested in the history of baby feeders, from pewter to ceramic to glass. Then followed pap boats and bubby pots.

Our interest in this hobby has enriched our appreciation of a wide range of medical history and it all stemmed from an early stage of my life in Gloucester as I began to explore the life of Dr Hadwen. Subsequently, as my interest was aroused in the sort of medication used and dispensed in Hadwen's time in a pharmacy and as a prescribing doctor I began to look into the subject a little further.

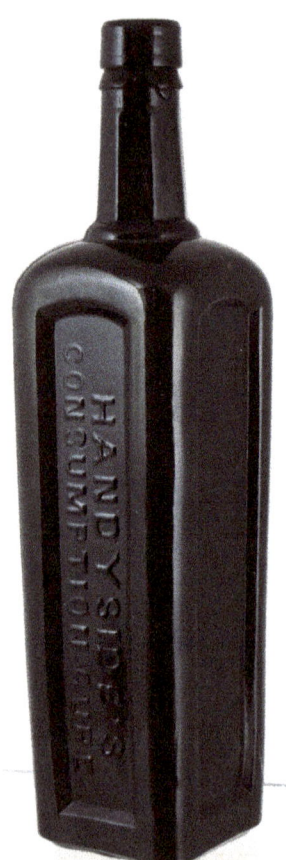

Handysides Consumption Cure also Handysides Rheumatic Cure Also Blood Purifier & Blood Food from Newcastle-upon-Tyne, famous for black glass medicine bottles

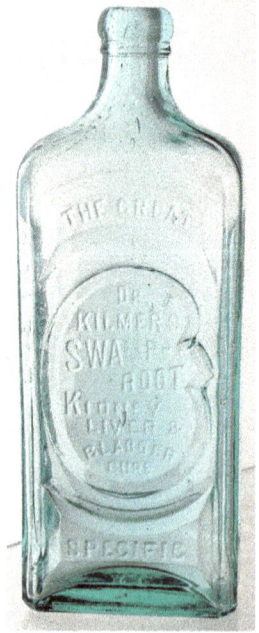

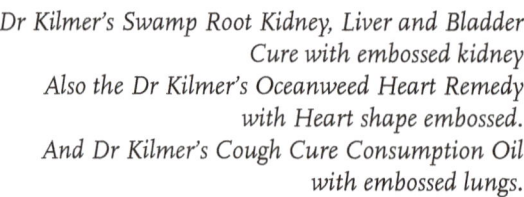

Dr Kilmer's Swamp Root Kidney, Liver and Bladder Cure with embossed kidney Also the Dr Kilmer's Oceanweed Heart Remedy with Heart shape embossed. And Dr Kilmer's Cough Cure Consumption Oil with embossed lungs.

15
SUCCESSION

This was the tribute printed in the *Citizen* newspaper on 31 December, 1932

> A generation has gone by since Dr Hadwen, then in early middle age, came to quicken this old controversy in the midst of a dire epidemic, and to establish for himself a position – unique and remarkable – as Hadwen of Gloucester, that will live on in the controversies, which veritably became the breath of life to him, long after his passing.

But time could not stand still.

Hadwen had been encouraged to seek a suitable assistant to work with him as he realised his health and energy were deteriorating. There is first hand knowledge of the association between Hadwen and Dr James Horsley. The latter was a graduate of Durham University in the 1920s and by this time was a vegetarian. In 1929 he helped Hadwen as a locum who eventually invited him to become his successor in the practice. In 1933, after Hadwen's death, Dr Horsley took over the practice. Those days were very different, and when enjoying a visit to the cinema but needed 'on call' his name would be projected onto the screen! Dr Horsley's wife states that the doctors did their own dispensing and the use of coloured aspirin tablets as a placebo was common. On the 'panel' or 'Club' cost three shillings and sixpence a week for a family, including medicines. Three to five shillings were charged for a home visit. A chauffeur was paid two pounds a week and he sometimes also acted as a receptionist.

Dr Horsley was a conscientious objector, and therefore was able to continue practising in Gloucester and during the war looked after patients whose family doctors had been drafted. He became the President of the Vegetarian Society and was opposed to inoculation.

His principles were compassion and gentleness to man and creature alike. He was a Trustee of the 'Order of the Cross' founded in 1904 as a Christian based group with the objectives of 'Informal fellowship for development of spiritual understanding of love and wisdom in life.'

Dr Horsley was the Family Doctor of Sir Stafford Cripps, former Chancellor of the Exchequer, who was a vegetarian by conviction on health grounds and also ethical reasons. They became friends and he accompanied Sir Stafford Cripps to Switzerland where Cripps was receiving treatment. Accurate detail is not known but it is possible Cripps had colitis.

Dr Horsley practised in Gloucester for over 40 years. He had suffered all his life with asthma. He died suddenly playing golf in 1965. A memorial service at St. Barnabas Church, Gloucester, was attended by over 500 people.

Dr Donald Morris was educated at Wycliffe College where he remembers Hadwen preaching a sermon in their chapel. He qualified in Medicine at St. Bartholomew's Hospital in London. He was a vegetarian and conscientious objector and chose to join as a partner after doing a locum for the practice in 1942. 1947 was the year of bad flooding and patients were visited by using a punt in lower Westgate, Dr Morris also delivered a baby in a filthy longboat on the docks.

By 1949 Dr John Campbell joined the partnership after National Service in the RAF, having qualified at Glasgow University. He also was a vegetarian. His special interest was orthopaedics.

Dr Margery van Zyl, a graduate of Aberdeen University, had knowledge of the partners of the day and shared their vegetarian habit and respect for animal life. She had the opportunity to observe and work in the practice as a medical student and then, when Dr Horsley was ill, assisted the partnership in 1964. She

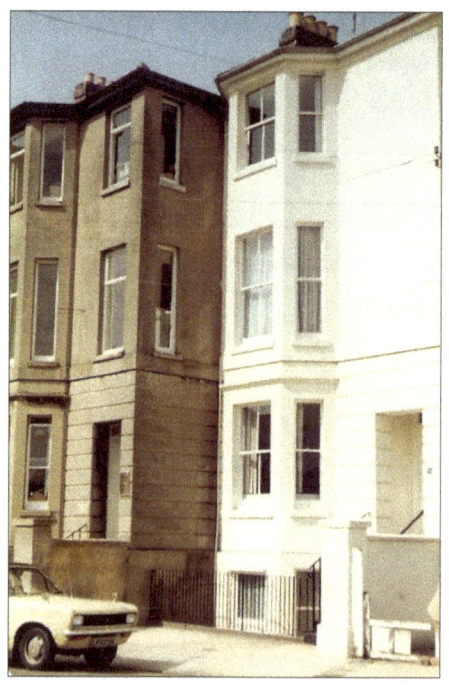

Premises at 25a Park Road

was invited to become a part-time partner in 1972. Margery had been friendly with Eulalie Rodenhust (Hadwen's granddaughter) for many years and once she decided to move to Gloucester with her two sons she was offered the opportunity to share accommodation at 'Hillside' along with Eulalie who had inherited the property from Hadwen.

This convenient arrangement continued for some years until a more suitable modern dwelling was purchased in Edge, near Stroud, where Margery lived with Eulalie until Eulalie died in 1997. This was then the last direct link with Hadwen's name and the practice.

By 1963 the partners had agreed to purchase the premises at 25a Park Road, overlooking the Gloucester Park. The basement and ground floor and part of the second floor provided consulting and reception areas. For many years a room was preserved for the use of members of the 'Order of the Cross' which included Drs Morris, Campbell and van Zyl and their families and associates to meet, and in particular hold a service on a Sunday morning.

Until 1970 the tradition and beliefs that Hadwen started were continued by the partners who held similar views and were vegetarians. This brief summary of the sequence of events after Hadwen's death is relevant to complete the story. Succeeding assistants and partners were appointed but not judged on their habits or convictions, solely on their suitability and experience that would enhance the services offered to patients.

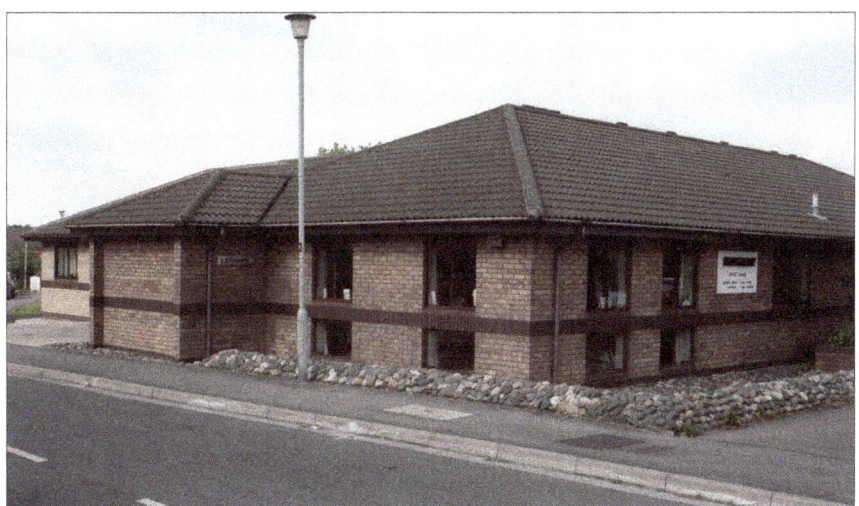

Initial development at Abbeydale, Glevum Way Surgery

From that time, as partners retired, changes inevitably took place and the practice continued to prosper. Patient numbers increased and extended facilities provided for more consultation areas, staff and reception, clinics and also the advent of the practice nurses. Antenatal and baby clinics with full immunisation programmes and also minor operation sessions were all part of new services offered to patients. The meeting room on the second floor was vacated and used as a consulting room with additional facilities. The top floor became designated as a flat for the use of trainees, for a year or so, working to gain experience. Permission was obtained to break through into the adjoining ground floor building to create even more space.

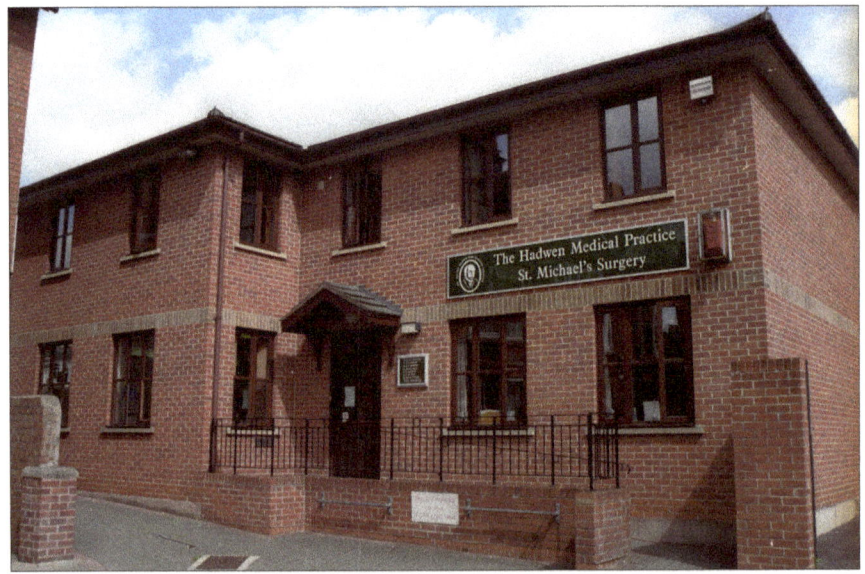

St. Michael's Square Surgery

However as General Medical Practice developed, services increased and housing development in the city also increased dramatically and better facilities were required.

Firstly, in 1984 a new purpose built surgery was constructed in the 'commercial zone' of the Abbeydale development and once this surgery was established, an opportunity arose to provide new premises in the city Centre. A site became available, just to the rear of 25a Park Road. By 1987 this new building was complete.

It became more common for partnerships to choose a name rather than be known by the senior partner of the day and various suggestions

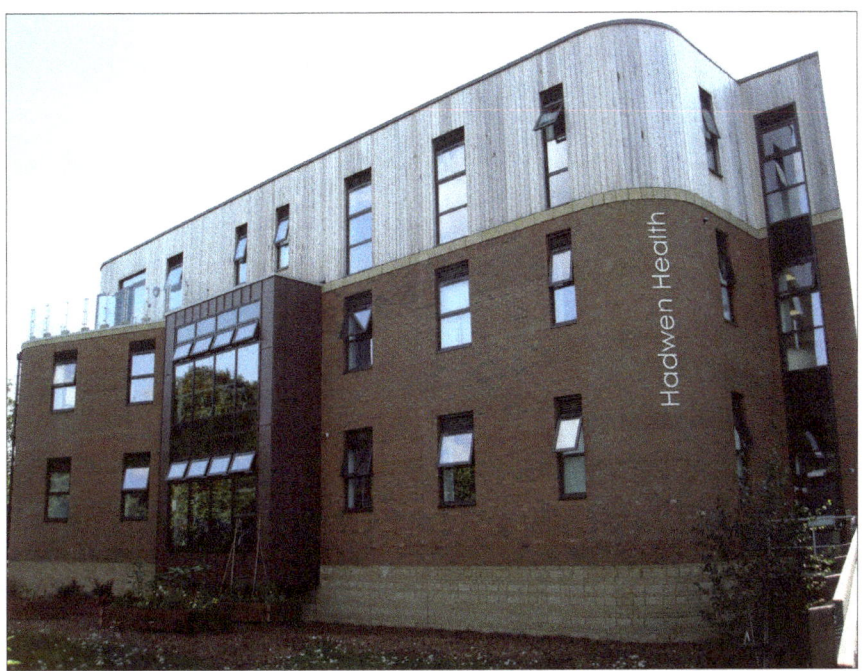

The new extension in Abbeydale which has become the hub of the practice serving an ever increasing population in the area

were put to the staff to vote for a suitable title and the result was that we were named 'The Hadwen Medical Practice'.

Finally, to complete the story, very recently (2018) a fine new extension has been completed adjoining the Glevum Way Surgery and the present partners have decided to continue to use the title with a little modification to 'Hadwen Health'.

The new extension in Abbeydale has become the hub of the practice serving an ever increasing population in the area.

16
POSTSCRIPT AND REFLECTIONS

SOME PATIENTS recorded their memories:-

Mr S. wrote he remembered Hadwen as a tall man riding a black bicycle to visit the house and also the queues of patients both up the surgery steps, and out down the street, waiting to be seen. Two pence for a bottle of medicine, from a stock supply, shaken in front of the patient with the instruction ' Take this three times a day, the gate swings long on a rusty hinge'. He remembered how strong the feeling was in Gloucester of support for Hadwen at the time of his trial. Mounted police had to hold the crowds back. He records he heard from Hadwen's housekeeper that after returning home after his visits he told her to send his lunch down the road to a patient who needed it more than he did.

Mrs B. visited Hadwen's house in Brunswick Square for afternoon tea. She was only a little girl and went there with her mother. Hadwen was kind and stopped to explain things to his patients about their illness. She wanted her sons to be vaccinated but her mother 'didn't believe it'. She quotes Hadwen saying 'vaccination was only given to pigs and animals'. She stated neither she nor her sister were vaccinated nor her seventeen grandchildren or nineteen great-grandchildren. Hadwen had signed a certificate to say that they should not be vaccinated.

Mr H. records that when he was ten years old his younger brother caught the 'so called smallpox' but never went to the isolation hospital and was not very ill. He and his elder brother then caught it and were taken off by ambulance to Brockworth aerodrome which had been turned into an isolation hospital. By this time the spots had come out, not very severe and we were otherwise well. Our own clothes were removed and replaced with hospital clothing which was uncomfortable. After initial homesickness we played about quite happily in the surrounding grounds. He spent two weeks there and was submitted to potash baths, two at a time and they became quite brown. Initially they could only speak to visitors through a high fence but later his father was given a white coat and allowed to make contact. Men and boys were separated from mothers and children. His brother went home first as he had been vaccinated but he had not, due to the influence of Dr Hadwen. The weather was very warm, we had sweets in our lockers and we were plagued with wasps. Apparently only the serious cases had suffered pockmarks. He remembered the word Alastrim being mentioned as a description of the disease.

Mr F. was fourteen years old when he was employed as a milk delivery boy carrying two large buckets of milk and measures on the handlebars of his bike. he had been vaccinated but his employer insisted he be revaccinated because he came into contact with so many customers. He wore a red armband to stop people knocking into his sore swollen arm. Some customers would not come to the door but left their jug by the door with cash in saucer containing disinfectant where he also placed any change. Brockworth aerodrome was nicknamed 'Pimple Town'

Miss H. living in London she sought a new post and at interview she was told she would have to be vaccinated as she came from Gloucester. She had to pay a doctor in Kensington five shillings to be 'done'. On returning to Gloucester she saw Dr Hadwen and he told her if she had gone to him sooner he would have got all the vaccine out. She was the only one out of nine siblings to be vaccinated. Her sister remembered in 1923 the chicken pox/ smallpox scare. Their bedrooms were shared, they were not ill with only a few spots and there was no need for them to go to 'Pimple Palace' at Brockworth. Visitors went out there to watch them playing in the fields. None of the family were vaccinated and her mother paid two shillings and sixpence at the police station to get a form signed not to have her child vaccinated. This certificate had to be signed before the child was six weeks old and a doctor had to sign it.

Mrs W. in 1923 was 13 years old and they had to go to Mary de Crypt Church to be vaccinated and then had to wear a a red armband. She was very fortunate as the vaccination did not take, so she didn't suffer pain like the others. She was told that she would never get smallpox.

Mrs B. states that her mother recalled the 1923 outbreak and her visits to people in isolation at the Gloucester and Cheltenham Factory at Brockworth where visitors stood back from the fence to talk to them. Her mother's sister-in-law was pregnant and as her own father was supposed to have smallpox at the time, no-one would look after her, so her mother visited every day to attend her.

Mr S. had 'smallpox' and spent two months at the Brockworth facility.

Mrs M. has a photograph of her aunt as Dr Hadwen's chauffeuse. She also remembered the distressing pamphlets posted through letter boxes showing the cruelty to live calves when lymph was extracted. Her mother was a Dr Hadwen supporter as, when she was young, she and her cousin were vaccinated and subsequently both developed psoriasis and people thought it was catching. Her cousin was so affected she could not be seen helping her husband as a bar tender and eventually committed suicide. It was thought they had been vaccinated with a dirty needle. Her mother remained healthy, with fifteen children, five being stillborn. The daughters did not have obvious psoriasis but two had to have inoculations to travel abroad and both had rashes as a result.

Patients paid tribute to his kindness and he even assisted in helping a wife, whose husband had gone to serve in the Great War. For three years he checked her weekly accounts and writing business letters for her so that she could carry on as usual until her husband returned.

The era of Dr Hadwen's life and achievements began to fade from memory but one further development took place to recognise his life's work. In 1970 the BUAV co-operated with other supporters in the founding of the 'Dr Hadwen Trust for Humane Research'; the objective was to find alternatives to animal experiments which succeeding Governments had insisted were justified in the need for medical research.

By the millennium the Registered Charity had income over five years of £800,000 for non-animal research projects. Patrons were Joanna Lumley OBE and David Shepherd OBE. Other named supporters are John Humphrys, Angela Rippon, Rory Bremner, Alan Titchmarsh, and Dame Judy Dench. The Charity research covers cancer, heart disease, arthritis, and meningitis without causing a single animal to suffer. In 2017 the Charity decided to have a new look to convey its purpose and a working name. It is now known as 'Animal Free Research UK'. It is still reported that four million animals are used in medical research in UK per annum.

Having paid due deference to Hadwen and his principles the reader might wonder where I stand in trying to give an overall view of this member of the medical profession, and so far have mainly avoided using much in the way of my own personal fascination with the story.

To a certain extent our lives have been interwoven, but not necessarily agreeing with all of Hadwen's convictions.

Firstly, I must state that no person can have a better start in life than to have had parents who were descendants of an established Lancashire family. I have included a small part of the Hadwen Family

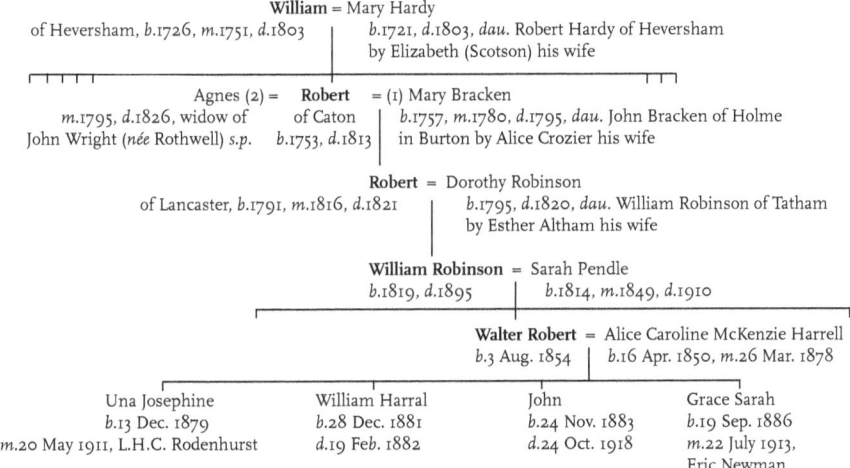

Tree, which is part of a comprehensive document showing relatives distributed around the northern area of Lancaster and the attractive Lune Valley. I am familiar with many of the villages from which they appear to originate and to my surprise this includes one relative who actually lived in my own village of Caton. (See 'Robert *born* 1753').

My upbringing was in a strict non-conformist family and alcohol was never allowed in the house. I have remained a teetotaller all my life in common with Hadwen.

I was educated at Lancaster Royal Grammar school and it is much to my annoyance that despite several enquiries I have been unable to confirm Kidd's statement that the grandfather of Walter was a pupil there.

Just as Hadwen, whilst living in Highbridge, had travelled to remote communities to preach or take part in Bible study, so was my experience to be aware that local Methodist ministers and lay preachers went out to speak at gatherings held in farmers' accommodation as their occupation and remoteness would restrict their opportunity to regularly attend the local chapel services.

In my first years at University I lived in student accommodation very close to Bedford Square and Bloomsbury where Hadwen lived and worked for a short time. Later, as a Medical Student living in a flat in Victoria, I cycled or bussed along Whitehall from Victoria and often looked at the facade of the anti-vivisection offices (see image chapter 13) and wondered why it was there in that situation. Now I know!

During my final year as a student there was the well publicised outbreak of Smallpox in Bradford and a close acquaintance of mine had been appointed to Bradford as a Consultant Pathologist. His colleague was in contact with a case which, initially, was not diagnosed definitively as 'smallpox'. The diagnosis was confirmed and the colleague declared he had never been vaccinated. He died very shortly after being exposed to the infected patient. The media highlighted the case and many people had not been vaccinated or had no record of such protection and a long queue formed in the street outside my hospital, all waiting for vaccination.

Once qualified I gained extra hospital experience working in the Woolwich area for a year, again following Hadwen's footsteps.

Eventually I arrived in Gloucester to join the Practice in 1969 and over a few years held Office in the BMA Gloucester Branch, eventually elected a Fellow. This is where our professional lives diverged and I doubt Hadwen would have approved. Not only that, but beginning to be interested in medical history, I became associated with the Jenner Museum in Berkeley, Gloucestershire. One of the supporters was Professor R. Shooter CBE, who investigated the last case of smallpox in UK. The infection had originated in the research laboratory at Birmingham University. Professor Shooter lived nearby and we met on several occasions. He provided a lot of material on the subject of smallpox for the Museum including examples of smallpox vaccination certificates from many countries.

Much later, once retired, we were holidaying in Northumberland and by chance saw a sign to Chillingham Castle which we followed into a forested area and eventually into a clearing where the castle stood. At that stage, I could only vaguely remember the historical visit recorded of Hadwen's short stay there but we were able to view most of the rooms open to the public. There followed a chance to book a viewing of the 'White Cattle' in the afternoon. We arrived at the gate which secured the cattle enclosure and awaited the warden's arrival. It appeared that we were the only visitors and so he invited us to join him in his farm vehicle as long as we did not wind down windows or attempt to touch the cattle. It was a privilege to sit surrounded by the cattle who were unperturbed and hardly inquisitive. We were given all the information about the breeding habits of the the herd. I corresponded with the present owner, Sir Humphry Wakefield. Bt. and provided a copy of Hadwen's record of his visit to Chillingham which may aid his efforts to restore the Castle in keeping with the original description.

IN ATTEMPTING to portray the life of Dr Hadwen as accurately as possible, I have tried to avoid my opinions being expressed but to stick to the facts available. I am glad to report that the practice flourishes and over the years modern medical practice has progressed. All families and services are available for patients and the bias amongst some patients against vaccination, still obvious in my early years in Gloucester, has gradually receded.

Animal experimentation and cruelty has received wide publicity over the years to the extent that the use of animals, in particular of primates, in laboratory investigation has been severely curtailed.

The question of the use of vaccination/immunisation procedures and their safety continues to be debated. There is 'herd complacency' resulting in reduced 'herd immunity' and, this in turn, places populations at risk of disease spread. People with reduced immune response are particularly put in danger. The so called 'Antivaxx' movement and 'false news' is part of a campaign that causes uncertainty and confusion amongst the public. The latter are ill-equipped to sort out the truth of the effectiveness of WHO health programmes.

There is no denying the success of smallpox vaccination in eradicating the world of this highly infectious and dangerous disease (1980). The worldwide campaign to similarly conquer poliomyelitis started in 1985 and is a much more complex problem. WHO alongside Rotary International, later joined by the Bill and Melinda Gates Foundation are slowly winning the battle with only one or two pockets of the virus in remote areas which is being carefully monitored. Final success in seeing the end of the second most infectious and damaging disease in the world is within reach. I would love to see smallpox and poliomyelitis be a problem of the past in my lifetime.

APPENDICES

I
Hadwen and Inquest and Charge of Manslaughter, as reported in *Gloucester Journal* 13th September 1924

THE ADJOURNED INQUEST into the circumstances attending the death of Nellie Christobelle Burnham, the ten and a half year old daughter of George Burnham, a steel presser, working in America, and Mrs Burnham, of 49, Vauxhall Rd, Gloucester, who died on 10 August was resumed at the Gloucester Petty Sessions on Friday afternoon by the city Coroner (Mr G Trevor-Wellington)

The coroner was accompanied by the Deputy Coroner (Dr J. A. Bell). Mr Percy Haddock (Cheltenham) represented the parents, Mr A. F. Clements (instructed by Messrs Langley-Smith and Son) appeared for Dr W. R. Hadwen: and Inspector T. A. James watched the proceedings on behalf of the police. Mr G. Newth was the foreman of the jury.

At the previous hearing on 13 August evidence was given by Ann Maria Burnham, the mother of the child, to the effect that on 1 August she called in Dr W. R. Hadwen to treat the child, who had a bad throat and talked thickly. The doctor saw the child again on 4 August and 9 August the mother alleging that on the latter occasion although Dr Hadwen said the child's throat was clearing nicely, she was much worse. Subsequently her brother-in-law called in Dr E. S. Ellis, who said the child was suffering from diphtheria and pneumonia and that there was little hope of her living. The child died the following day. Dr Ellis also gave evidence as to his diagnosis, and stated that diphtheria was not difficult to diagnose and by taking a swab it could be diagnosed with accuracy. Dr Ellis said he thought that the proper treatment and accurate diagnosis ought to have saved the child's life.

The inquest was resumed on 14 August but adjourned owing to the absence of witnesses abroad.

At the outset of the proceedings Mr Clements asked that he might be allowed to ask a few questions of the mother.

The Coroner said he would recall her.

Her previous evidence having been read over, Mrs Burnham, in reply to Mr Clement's questions, said that on the Saturday previous to the child's death she gave the deceased milk as ordered by Dr Hadwen. The last time deceased vomited was on Friday. Before she died the girl was drowsy all the day, as she had been all the time she had been ill. This intensified on the Saturday. Before midnight Dr Ellis injected something witness did not see, and she died later. The girl was not getting better on the previous Wednesday and witnesses did not tell anyone that she was going on nicely on that day. She did not remember anything that she was told by Dr Hadwen on the Wednesday that would be likely to make the child worse or liable to pneumonia. On Thursday night when she went across the road at the neighbours, the deceased got out of bed and went downstairs in her bare feet for water. A little brother gave her the water to drink.

Mr Clements:- Did you tell anyone about it?

Witness:- Yes, I told a neighbour

Mr Clements:- Was it Mr Tanner?

Witness:- No

Mr Clements:- Did Mr Tanner say it was enough to cause the child's death?

Witness:- No, the child was back in bed in a few minutes. She was comfortable when I returned home.

Mr Clements:- Did you tell Dr Ellis about the incident?

Witness:- No

Mr Clements:- Why not?

Witness:- I was worried at the time and did not think about it.

Mr Clements:- Did Mr Tanner ask you on 2 September if you had told the doctor about the incident?

Witness:- No

At this point the coroner ordered all the witnesses except the medical ones to leave the court, in view of the turn the cross-examination had taken.

Mr Clements:- Have you ever told Mr Tanner that you did not tell the doctor, and that you intended to keep it to yourself?

Witness:- No, he is a liar.

Mr Clements:- Did Mr and Mrs Tanner say it was not fair to the doctors not to mention it?

Witness:- Neither of them mentioned it.

The Coroner:- Did Dr Hadwen explain to you what position the child should be kept in?

Witness:- No.

The Coroner:- That you were to keep her still and in a recumbent position?

Witness:- No

Answering further questions, witness said her daughter Hilda, aged eighteen was in Over Hospital suffering from diphtheria. Dr Hadwen had not seen this girl. Her daughter, Gladys (aged four years) was attended by Dr Hadwen on 12 August. She was still in hospital with nasal diphtheria. Olive Cornock, a little girl who was a relation of the neighbour, had played with witness's daughter Gladys on 9 August. She was removed to hospital on 12 August.

Answering Mr Haddock witness said that all the children had evidence of nasal discharge similar to that the deceased child had.

Dr Hadwen saw them and said Leonard, a son, had an ulcerated throat.

Matilda Taylor, wife of Ernest Taylor, an electrical fitter, 82 Ladysmith Rd, said the deceased was her niece. She first saw her during her illness, on 9 August at 9.30 am. Witness thought the child very ill. She took milk with difficulty. Witness was present when Dr Hadwen came in at 10.30 am. The previous witness told him that she thought the child was worse and very weak. Dr Hadwen sounded her chest and felt her pulse, and said there was scarcely anything the matter with the child and that she would soon be alright. The doctor looked down the child's throat and said it was clearing nicely. He told the mother to give the child plenty of cold milk. He was told that the child could not take the medicine ordered and Dr Hadwen told the mother to put a little water with it. The doctor was there about five minutes. Witness left the house at about eleven o'clock and went back at 7.30pm. She could see that the child was much worse. There was a consultation among the members of the family and Dr Ellis was called. Witness was with the child from the time Dr Ellis called until the child died. Deceased tried to vomit about quarter of an hour before she died.

Albert Austen Fudge, foreman fitter of 54 Bury Road, Saltley, Birmingham said the deceased was his niece. He saw her on 7 August when he thought she was very ill. She had a green discharge from her nose, tinged with red. He did not see her until after 9pm on the following Saturday when following a family conference he telephoned Dr Hadwen telling him he did not think the treatment he was giving the little girl was good enough, and that the family had decided to call in another doctor. Dr Hadwen said he had done his best and rang off.

By Mr Clements:- Dr Hadwen did not say that it was a 'free country' and that they could have any doctor they desired. Mrs Burnham had not told him that the child had gone down stairs in her bare feet on the Wednesday or Thursday night.

Sarah Jane Peachey, wife of William Peachey, 47 Vauxhall Rd said she first saw the child, who was always strong and healthy on 4 August in bed. She was very ill and had a running discharge from eyes, nose and mouth, tinged with blood and there was an offensive smell. She told the mother that she believed it to be diphtheria. Witness saw the girl on 9 August at two pm when she was very much worse. Witness was not surprised when she said the girl was dead the next morning.

Dr Ellis was next recalled and his previous evidence having been read in answer to Mr Haddock said that when he examined the child's throat he used a tongue depressor, at the end of which was an electric lamp, so that he had a good light at the back of the throat. He gave the child no injection of any sort.

By the Coroner:- Diphtheria was a common complaint which needed careful watching as sudden changes were apt to take place, by which the patient's progress could be determined. Strain on the heart had to be looked for, which could be discovered by use of the stethoscope and the pulse. In hospital the pulse would be taken not less frequently than every four hours and in private practice there should be frequent visits.

The Coroner:- Would the case be adequately attended where there was a larger lapse of a day?

Witness:- No

Dr Ellis said it might be difficult to distinguish between diphtheria and follicular tonsillitis. Temperature did not matter much in the latter disease, but the pulse rate was of some importance. An offensive smell characterised diphtheria, but it was to be found in follicular tonsillitis. He did not think the incident of walking downstairs did not necessarily prejudice the child's chance of recovery.

By Mr Clements:- It was unlikely the incident led to pneumonia but it might have done. It was possible for an experienced medical man to make a mistake as to diphtheretic membrane.

Mr Clements:- could you make the mistake?

Witness:- Yes, but I did not.

Dr Ronald Briers Berry, the city Medical Officer of Health, stated he had received no notification of diphtheria at 49, Vauxhall Rd from Dr Hadwen. He received a notification from Dr Ellis on 11 August in respect of the deceased. On 12 August he received from Dr Graham a notification of diphtheria in respect of Helen Burnham, aged eighteen years but she was removed to hospital the previous day on a telephone notification. He had treated her, and the attack had been a fairly severe one. On 12 August there was a notification of a case of doubtful diphtheria from Dr Ellis in regard to Olive Cornock aged seven years of 27 Widden St, who had been at the Burnham's house the previous week. She was removed to hospital and discharged on Friday last. A notification of diphtheria in regard to Gladys, aged four years, was made as a result of a visit to the house by witness's assistant, Dr Colquhoun. The attack was a fairly severe one and she was still in hospital under witness' care.

By Mr Haddock:- He agreed that the pulse rate was important in diagnosing diphtheria. He thought it was possible to distinguish between offensive smell caused by diphtheria and tonsillitis.

By Mr Clements:- He should not accept the filing of a positive swab as proof of diphtheria, he would look at all the symptoms.

The Coroner:- Looking at the case of the deceased clinically, as Dr Hadwen had appeared to have done, ought diphtheria to have been suspected?

Witness:- Yes.

By the exercise of competent skill and sufficient attention ought diphtheria to have been diagnosed and treated?

Witness:- Yes, on general principles.

Mr Clements:- Do you express any opinion as to the time that could have been done?

Witness:- That would depend upon the time that membrane was there.

Mr Clements:- That would be the deciding factor?

Witness:- Yes, in the clinical diagnosis.

Mr Clements:- If there had been no membrane present when Dr Hadwen examined, could he have dismissed diphtheria as out of the question?

Witness:- Not altogether.

Mr Clements:- Suppose there was no membrane, no blood in the nasal discharge, and other children getting better, would that justify the doctor deciding against diphtheria

Witness:- Not altogether.

Dr William Washbourn stated that he made a post mortem examination in the presence of Dr Bell, on 12 August. The body was poorly nourished and there was a puncture of the skin at the back of the chest on the right side which was sealed by a dressing. The back of the throat, the tonsils, the soft palate, the larynx were intensely inflamed and congested, so much so that the mucus membrane was in one or two places almost black. there was a patch of adherent membrane on the back of the epiglottis. there was acute congestion of the trachea and bronchial tubes on both sides. The left lung was inflated, but the right lung was solid throughout from inflammation. The right bronchial tubes in addition to congestion were almost completely filled with dense membrane, some of which was adherent and had evidently been formed where found, but above the adherent portion there was a piece of loose membrane, which had apparently been inhaled from higher up. The right pleural cavity contained two to three fluid ounces of clear fluid. the heart was healthy, as were other organs. Death in his opinion was due to the diphtheria and pneumonia.

By Mr Haddock:- The absence of membrane visible from the mouth was not inconsistent with what Dr Ellis had stated. It might have separated during the last hour of life. The loose patch might have been part of what Dr Ellis saw. If there were membrane present on Saturday night, it must have been present on Saturday morning. From post mortem appearance it had been in existence two or three days. Taking the pulse rate would help diagnosis even in a doubtful case. Blood tinged nasal discharge would give rise to suspicion of diphtheria even without the presence of membrane. The presence of an offensive smell would make it more suspicious, the smell in diphtheria was extremely characteristic. From the clinical symptoms, and the conditions of the other 3 children, and leaving bacteriology out of the question, a medical man should have been at least highly suspicious that the case was diphtheria.

Answering Mr Clements, Dr Washbourn said if there had been no membrane, and no blood in the discharge, it would make it less likely that it was diphtheria. It was not a fact that membrane was always present in diphtheria. It was possible to mistake membrane for other things. The loose piece of membrane might have come from the larynx.

The incident of the child going down stairs might have resulted in a chill from which a sudden attack of pneumonia might arise. The child had sufficient pneumonia to cause death, but he did not think it caused death by the adherent membrane in the bronchial tubes. It was not possible to say for certain whether the child died from the pneumonia or not.

By the Coroner:- In a diphtheria case sufficient attention could not be given by missing a day in the visits.

The coroner said that he proposed to call Dr Hadwen subject to the usual caution.

Mr Clements intimated that the doctor would give evidence.

The coroner said he anticipated so.

Mr Clements said he would first like the neighbour Tanner to be recalled.

The Coroner agreed.

George Henry Tanner, painter, 44, Vauxhall Rd, said he remembered Mrs Burnham telling him on 6 August on his asking how the child was, that the doctor had been that morning and the child was much better. On the following night, Mrs Burnham said, while standing at the door of his house, that the child had got out of bed, came downstairs, and went to the scullery for water. He said it was enough to cause the child's death, and she replied that it was a bad sign. Subsequently in witness' house he asked Mrs Burnham if she intended to let the doctor know, and she had said she had not, and that it was her own business. He felt it was his duty, on reading the evidence in the newspaper at the beginning of the inquest, and feeling that half the evidence of Mrs Burnham was false, to tell Dr Hadwen, and he gave a written statement to Mr W. Langley-Smith.

The Coroner:- Did it not occur to you that it was your duty to go to the coroner or to his officer.

Witness:- I did not know then.

Coroner:- Do you know Dr Hadwen?

Witness:- Yes

Coroner:- Well?

Witness:- No

Coroner:- If you thought it was your duty to assist in the administration of justice, why did you not go to the office of Justice?

Witness:- I did not know where that was.

By Mr Haddock:- Other statements that were false were that child was worse on Wednesday and that she called in Dr Ellis.

At this point, there was an adjournment for half an hour.

Dr Walter Robert Hadwen entered the witness box, and having been sworn in and was told by the Coroner that he needed answer no question which would commit him. He said he held degrees of MD MRCS and LRCP. He was trained in Bristol Hospital and St. Bartholomew's.

He had practised about 35yrs, 28 yrs of which had been in Gloucester and he had a long experience of diphtheria and other infectious diseases. On 21 July he was called to see Leonard Burnham and treated him for ulcerated tonsillitis. He considered the question of diphtheria but he was decidedly of the opinion it was not that disease. There was not a vestige of membrane on the uvula and soft palate. There was no nasal discharge or foul breath. and the mother said nothing about either. He prescribed a saline mixture and gargle of vinegar and hot water, which was his sheet anchor for sore throat and which he had used with success in thousands of cases. He was called to Gladys (aged four) who had a slight attack of tonsillitis but no symptoms of diphtheria.

On 1 August he was called to see the deceased. She had a bad cold and a watery discharge from the nose, but there was no blood present. The mother said nothing about it. There was no offensive smell. He examined her to see if diphtheria were present but her condition was the same as the other children. There were no symptoms of diphtheria. On the first day he saw her she had ulcer spots on the tonsils and she had ulcerated tonsillitis. He prescribed an expectorant medicine because she had bronchial catarrh with a suspicion of bronchial pneumonia and a similar gargle as for the other child. He saw her again on the following Monday when the ulcer spots had coalesced and contracted. On Wednesday the spots on the right tonsil were only small, and on the other they were shrivelled. There was no membrane present. On his first visit he told the mother that the girl's throat looked like a scarlet fever throat but after a careful examination he dismissed the possibility of scarlet fever. On the Wednesday he advised the continuance of the mixture and the use of the gargle, and the mother said the girl could not get the gargle back far enough into the throat. He therefore told her to get some pure glycerine and paint the back of the throat. He used glycerine because it was an excellent solvent of all membrane. He had used it in scores of cases with success. He gave a general denial to the statement of the mother that he was never longer in the house for more than five minutes and what she had described him as doing on the last visit would of necessity take five minutes. He felt the child's pulse every time he went to the house. He usually looked at the throat and took the pulse at the same time. On the first occasion he took the pulse to see if there was any fever because the child had bronchial catarrh. On the same occasion he took the deceased temperature and it was 100 degrees, the mother was present. It gave him no anxiety whatever and he told the mother the child would be well in a few days.

Up to Wednesday there was no symptoms present to indicate diphtheria. As to her general condition on Wednesday, 6 August, the deceased was sitting up and smiling and very much better. The mother told him the child was very much better and getting on nicely before he saw the child. The pulse was normal, the throat had cleared with the exception of one spot, and with the exception of being week, the child was practically well. He told the mother that the child should have a tonic and he prescribed a syrup of the phosphate mixture. The glands in the neck were not affected, whereas every genuine case of diphtheria had been characterised by large sub-maxillary glands and square jaw. He saw nothing to suggest diphtheria in any one of the children from the first to the last. If membrane had been present he would have seen it. On Saturday 9 August, he said to the mother that the throat had cleared up nicely, meaning that the ulceration had gone. It was quite easy to diagnose diphtheria – in fact there was nothing easier in this world. The membrane could not be mistaken and had it been there he would have seen it. He did not take a swab because diphtheria bacillus was found in every kind of sore throat and in the majority of healthy throats.

The Coroner:- do you really mean that?

Witness:- I say there are the germs in your throat now

Witness proceeding, said there was no clinical symptoms or physical signs of diphtheria in the deceased from first to last. On Saturday, August 9th, before her death, he was taken aback by the marked change in the child. He questioned the mother. He examined the throat and there was no vestige of membrane present, there was no blood discharge and he noticed nothing in the way of offensive breath or he would have taken notice of these things. The trouble was inflammation of the right lung known as croupous pneumonia. He had intended to see the child the previous day, but owing to rush of business he had postponed the visit until Saturday. By the rules of the Club to which the parents of the deceased belonged they could call the doctor at any time in case of emergency.

On 9 August the mother said nothing about the incident of the child going downstairs. In view of the marked change, he tried to get the reason for the change from the mother but could not do so. The child was so bad that he did not prescribe medicine and he pressed the mother to give cold milk to keep the strength up. He told the mother it was the child's only chance. He never said to her that there was little or nothing the matter with the child. Such a suggestion was absurd. He left the house and the next he heard about the child was from the witness Fudge at 9pm that night over the telephone. The man said he was dissatisfied with witness's treatment and that he must have another doctor. Witness said that the child had been getting on very well until that day and Fudge said he did not agree and he was very dissatisfied. Witness said he had done his best for the child and Fudge said he would have another doctor in consultation otherwise witness would have welcomed a second opinion. Dr Hadwen said he next heard of the case on Wednesday 13 August at 3 o'clock, the day of the inquest an hour and a half before the opening.

The Coroner pointed out that he himself had tried to get in touch with the witness hours before that, but failed.

Witness proceeding: said that Dr Ellis had not communicated with him at all.

The Coroner said that would have been improper.

Mr Clements said that he meant before the death. There was no suggestion of unprofessional conduct. The Coroner said they were going outside the scope of the enquiry. Unless there was a definite charge being made, he should take notice of that.

Dr Hadwen added he had made up his mind to call on the Saturday evening but he did not do so after the telephone message. Witness did not attend the post mortem.

The Coroner said there was no obligation for the Coroner to invite a person to be present at a postmortem examination. Sometimes it was undesirable altogether.

Dr Hadwen said he was satisfied with the post mortem examination. Croupous or lobar pneumonia never followed diphtheria, for there was essential difference between that and lobular pneumonia which followed diphtheria.

The Coroner remarked that 3 doctors had been called and no question on this point had been put to them. Dr Hadwen said that the lobar pneumonia was a sudden attack and ending in the lung becoming solid, whilst lobular pneumonia inflammation was in patches and was of a progressive character. With regard to the separation of the membrane, witness held that the weakly condition of the child caused the vitality to be so low as to be impeded to throw off the membrane between the time of the visit by Dr Ellis until death. The use of the swab would not cause the separation of the membrane.

Mr Clements:- do you consider the action of the child in going downstairs to get the water brought on pneumonia? Witness: I do most decidedly. The child died from pneumonia and the post mortem showed that it was a stage of development of about 2 or 3 days.

Answering Mr Haddock, Witness, said he thought that the child's condition on August 9th was precarious, but he told the mother that he thought the child would pull through all right. He did not want to frighten the mother for that was not his habit. He denied the statement that he told the mother that there was nothing the matter with the girl. There was no need to tell the mother the child was seriously ill for the mother knew it. He denied that the child was suffering from diphtheria, in spite of the post mortem examination, or that it played a part in the death. When he said the throat was clear he meant that the ulcerated spots had gone but the throat was congested. The presence of membrane, adherent or loose, was indicative of lobar pneumonia. There were all kinds of membrane in the lungs which could not be distinguished from diphtheria membrane without bacteriological examination.

The Coroner:- can you give me an authority for that statement

Witness:- Yes, Osler's medicine a standard work, has a whole page devoted to the difference between diphtheroid and diphtheritic membranes.

Mr Haddock:- If you say you could recognise the diphtheritic membrane in the throat why should not Dr Washbourn recognise it in the larynx at the postmortem? Witness:- I cannot say

The Coroner:- But Dr Washbourn found the membrane and he isolated the bacillus? Witness:- He had not isolated the bacillus. He has taken it from the swab taken from the patient, which I would think was much better? What the postmortem showed was the membrane in the lungs not the throat.

Proceeding Dr Hadwen answering Mr Haddock, said that the fact the other 3 children were in hospital with diphtheria was a coincidence. On most points of opinion he disagreed in the case with Dr Ellis or Dr Washbourn. It was extraordinary that Dr Ellis diagnosed the case as diphtheria at once. He did not believe any medicine was of use in croupious pneumonia but on August 9th he was not sure about it being that disease. It was impossible to give the child medicine in its low state, but he would refuse to give child stimulants at any time. The only course was to give the child a fighting chance with plenty of milk. The girl had one good lung and with milk he thought she would pull through.

Replying to the Coroner, the witness said he saw nothing in the physical signs to justify asking the mother as to blood in the discharge from the nose. Mrs Burnham told him nothing about offensive breath.

The Coroner: do you maintain that the bacillus of diphtheria is to be found in even every healthy throat?

Witness:- in a great many.

The Coroner:-Do you agree that recent research has proved that to be a fallacy and that the bacillus formerly found was confused with another bacillus which has since been isolated?

Witness:- No

The Coroner:- It is the work of the Medical Research Council. Do you accept that as an authority?

Witness :- No It is the work of only one man.

The Coroner:- Pardon me but it is the work of a number of experts, selected by the Government.

Witness:-I should like to point out that the modern germ theory is all bosh.

The Coroner:-That is the only reasonable explanation for some of your evidence, that is your opinion.

Witness:- It is not a question of opinion. You made the statement with great emphasis that the bacillus was present in many healthy throats. The latest figures, even among contacts, where the percentage should be high, is only 8%? The matter is not worth arguing about. Bacteriology changes often like fashion

Replying to Mr Clements, Dr Hadwen said he agreed with eminent authorities like Professor Cruikshank and Osler in the views they held in regard to the diphtheria bacillus.

This concluded Dr Hadwen's statement which had occupied 2 hours.

Dr Washbourn was recalled and said Croupous pneumonia was not accompanied by the membrane he saw in the bronchial tubes and larynx at the postmortem examination. The membrane had the typical wash leather appearance described by Dr. Hadwen in his evidence.

In response to Mr Clements, witness stated that the pneumonia he found was the kind of pneumonia he would expect to find a child contracting after a sudden chill.

By the foreman of the jury: He did not think the child developed croupous pneumonia by coming downstairs, but she might have done.

Dr Ellis was also recalled, and in reply to a query by the jury, said he did not think the child contracted pneumonia by going downstairs, mainly because of the stage found at the postmortem. Nevertheless it may have begun there.

By Mr Clements: Croupous pneumonia would follow a sudden chill.

In his address to the jury, the coroner said that as to the facts they were the sole and unfettered judges. He pointed out the difference between negligence and crass negligence. Allegations had been made, and they had been denied. there had been allegations of a failure to diagnose and a failure to treat with competent skill and sufficient ability. Mr Wellington pointed out that there was a statuary obligation to notify diphtheria, but if, as Dr Hadwen believed, diphtheria did not exist, the point did not arise. If the jury thought there were any doubt, Dr Hadwen was entitled to it. If it were an error of judgement only, that might render him liable to civil liability but not criminal liability. There were several questions the jury had to ask themselves. The first was to decide whether diphtheria was the cause of death or not. The second was whether there was negligence by reason of failure to use competent skill and, or, give sufficient attention. If they thought there was negligence did they think it was gross? Finally, did they believe that the negligence caused, contributed to or accelerated the death of the deceased.

The jury retired to consider their verdict at about 9pm seven hours after the commencement of proceedings.

After an absence of nearly three quarters of an hour, the jury returned and the foreman handed in a written verdict, which he said was the verdict of nine of the 12 jurymen.

The verdict was that 'the child died from diphtheria and pneumonia and that Dr Hadwen failed to show competent skill and special attention, in consequence of which failure the child died.'

The Coroner: That in law, is a verdict of manslaughter, and therefore there must be a verdict accordingly. There must also be a committal.

Having asked Dr Hadwen to stand up, the Coroner said: "

Walter Robert Hadwen. I have no alternative but to commit you on my inquisition to take your trial at the next assizes for the city of Gloucester. There will be an application for bail?"

Mr Clements:- Yes

Mr Wellington said that under the state he did not think there was any power for him to accept Dr Hadwen in his own recognisance. The Coroner's act allowed him to accept sureties which he would do gladly. If he had the power to accept Dr Hadwen's personal recognisance he would do so without hesitation.

Mr Clements said he thought the Coroner could do so. The Coroner said there would be no difficulty in getting people in court to act as sureties. He would accept Dr Hadwen in £100 and 2 house holders in £25 each. Mr Langley-Smith "Cannot you take me in £500? The Coroner said it had been laid down by the Lord Chief Justice that a solicitor could not be bail for his own client.

Eventually Dr James Adamson Bell and Mr Alfred John Wiley 215 Barton St. Gloucester were accepted as sureties.

It is understood that Dr Hadwen will attend the Gloucester Police Station at 11. 30 am on Saturday morning. The hearing lasted nearly 8 hrs.

2
Premature Burial
Book by Tebb & Vollum
Second Edition Edited by Dr W. R. Hadwen
Published 1904 440 pages with illustrations

Fear of being buried alive is taphophobia (grave fear).

The advent of Cremation increased the public's fear of the misdiagnosis of death.

'It is true that hardly any one sign of death, short of putrefaction, can be relied upon as infallible.' BMJ 1885

I HAVE TRIED to summarise the salient point of this publication. This subject was described as the horror of the 19th century. Peculiarly, many articles were published on the subject in Germany and France but little in English publications until this book brought the whole subject, with references, to give a detailed summary of the topic. The only preventive measure for the individual (before death) is to make known their wish to have a postmortem or their jugular vein severed to be sure there was no sign of life or circulation. At the end of the 19th century people were still being buried without the necessary death certificate or even being examined by a doctor. Regulations limited the time to be taken between death and burial so as to reduce the risk of spreading disease. Therefore there was increased risk of premature burial in missing the diagnoses of coma, catalepsy or trance.

In epidemics, such as, plague, cholera and small-pox, errors in diagnosing "death' resulted in narrow escapes during such busy periods. There was a need to speed interment owing to the overcrowding of wards in hospitals and also of the mortuaries themselves. Also the great fear of disease being spread if burial was delayed.

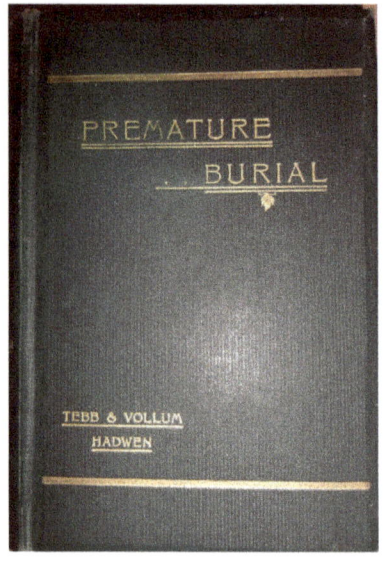

This book was presented to Dr. Till by a local Gloucester GP (Dr Watson) and was the first copy I had seen. I have never found a "first edition". New hardback editions are available on line!

Trance was variously described as 'Death Trance', 'Hysterical Trance', or 'Lethargic Trance'.

Egyptians had bodies supervised by priests before, later, embalming. The Greeks chopped off fingers before cremation to prove life extinct. Roman rulers likewise commanded that interment be delayed for a week or longer to ensure that death had occurred.

Holding a mirror to detect exhalation was a very inaccurate clinical sign of death. Described, also, is the use of a wine glass placed over the mouth and checked later for any sign of condensation.

Poultices were applied to chest and legs to stimulate (cause pain) and blister. Faradisation was used to ensure no response to muscle activity in a cadaver. Injections of sulphuric ether or other 'cocktail' of drugs were also tried to stimulate a response.

Multiple descriptions of potential premature deaths ensue with subsequent revival for many at the last moment. Modern medical terminology is rarely used in descriptions and scientific diagnosis cannot accurately be applied to the situation.

An exceptional instance is related:-

'The lady arrived from Senegal and was suspected of suffering from yellow fever and transferred to hospital under the care of the health officer. There, her condition worsened and she apparently died. The body became rigid and the face ashen and corpse like, and in that condition she was buried. The nurse, however, had noticed that the body was not cold, and that there was tremulousness of the muscles of the abdomen, and expressed the opinion that the patient had been prematurely buried. On this being reported a relative had the body exhumed, when it was found that a child had been born in the coffin. The autopsy showed the patient had not contracted yellow fever and had died of asphyxiation. The resulting legal action resulted in an £8, 000 damages being awarded.

Syncope, catatonic state, melancholia, hysteria are rather vague features to identify the problem causing death. Despite this, a challenge of suspected misadventure, misdiagnosis or possible poisoning rarely resulted in the authorities agreeing to exhumation.

A further chapter describes examples of torpidity, hibernation, suspended animation. Also the demonstration of the power of Fakirs from India to induce trance and mimic death for the public to witness and see recovery after many days after burial.

It seems that typical mistakes in death diagnosis occurred when people were struck by lightning or had evidence of alcohol excess apparently named as 'suspended animation'. Many apocryphal stories of premature burial are described by undertakers in their professional journal. Also stories by sextons and gravediggers.

Incidences of narrow escapes result in some individual being able to show their own death certificates issued in error! Those who survive a 'near death' experience can describe accurately all that was said by those in attendance and the discussions about funeral arrangements. Others remember nothing of their experience and are unaware of what has happened to them.

Another example relates that a lady experienced a shock or fright when 6 months pregnant and this brought on convulsions (? eclampsia) for 4hrs and then was thought to be dead. 5 attendant physicians agreed she was dead except one who demurred who applies a further painful stimulus after which there were minimal signs of life. Two days later she opens her eyes and had no recollection as to what had happened and then gave birth to a dead child. Thereafter she recovered her health completely.

The authors decry the delays and difficulties in gaining permission from Mayors, magistrates, sheriff or other officials, to open a grave or coffin when their is a suspected problem. Even delay in opening up vaults may have resulted in suffering and death when a person had been prematurely buried.

It was recognised that a patient who had suffered severe cold may be mistakingly thought to be dead but in a warmer atmosphere signs of life become evident. Misuse of early anaesthetic agents such as chloroform and other drugs such as digitalis and morphia may well have caused death to be diagnosed and no resuscitation attempts made. Religious practices which involve early burial or cremation (sometimes in public) may increase the risk of error without medical certification.

Wills expressed various wishes as to how death of the man involved should be ensured before burial. This even included a wish to have his head severed from his body by his nominated surgeon. Even Hans Christian Anderson carried a note in his pocket entreating his friends to make sure he was really dead before burial. The problem with wills and notes is that they may not come to light until after the funeral.

Evidence of decomposition should be observed before autopsy, embalming, cremation or burial, as a safeguard. This particularly should apply in cases of 'sudden death'.

There are descriptions of many clinical signs that can be taken as life extinction but many are fallible or misinterpreted. Much criticism is made of medical schools not even mentioning the deceptive nature of death and that the lack of compulsory personal medical inspection of the dead to certify the outcome should become law. Lax and perfunctory issuing of death certificates in hospitals was recognised as a problem when the body had neither been seen by the doctor or identified. In 1901, 10, 000 uncertified causes of death were recorded.

Whenever graveyards have been removed, as has happened in America where cities have expanded, unmistakeable evidence of premature burial have been disclosed.

The book continues with details of how the Law and Customs vary from country to country. Large sums of money have been bequeathed

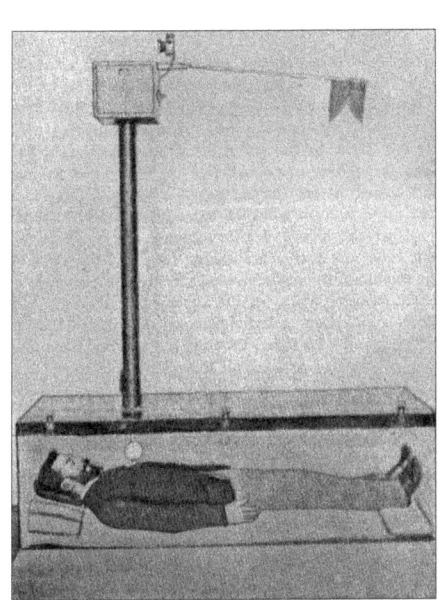 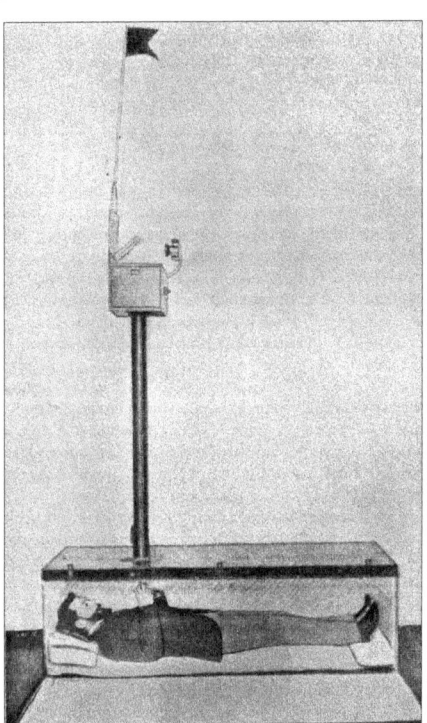

Body in Repose with system "set" *System "triggered"*
"Count Karnice-Karnicki's Invention"

by patrons to anyone who can document the discovery of a simple and common means of recognising, beyond doubt, the absolute signs of death, by such a test as could be adopted by poor villagers without technical instruction.

Count Karnice-Karnicki's invention is described with an airtight body box buried and a tube inserted in a sealed aperture to protrude above ground. If the person moves or breathes, a mechanism releases a spring which in turn activates a box mounted at the top of the tube which is designed to be tamper proof. The box lid then opens to allow air and some light into body chamber. At the same time a bell rings for half an hour (!!), a small flag rises perpendicularly and an electric lamp burns. the tube can act as a speaking tube. Cost of the apparatus was 12 shillings in 1901. The cemetery watchman (presumably there for such problems and to safeguard against body snatchers) would be alerted and raise the alarm. Many similar devices were produced.

The subject of Premature Burial continued throughout Europe and America and there were sensational publications in many newspapers and 'confirmed' reports in medical press of 'came to Life' and 'return to life'. Described is the case of a man supposedly dead for 24hrs, the body was cold and he had suffered apoplexy. He was wrapped and sewn up in his funeral shroud and left till the time of the burial, but on the way to the cemetery the bearers heard muffled noises within the coffin which was accordingly opened, three medical men who were passing were appealed to in order to pronounce on the man's condition. Restorative means were employed and in a few days he was well.

What then developed were 'Waiting Mortuaries' where, in Germany in particular, bodies were deposited until putrefaction was evident. In France there were appointed in every district a 'medical inspector of the dead' and to give a formal certificate. Thereafter the body could be removed.

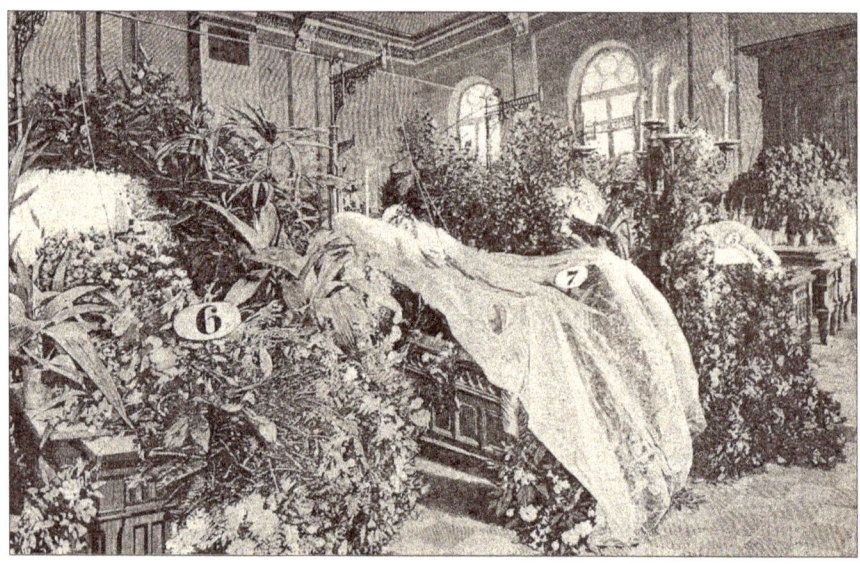

A Waiting Mortuary, as described. Note the numbering, the sloping slabs on which the bodies were mounted and the cord and pulley system can be seen. Flower arrangements were provided as part of the service. The body is labelled with a ticket. Temperature and ventilation are controlled. There is a caretaker who makes inspections routinely and is alerted by any bell ringing. A further medical examination then takes place before interment.

Munich had 10 fine mortuaries built, replete with every modern appliance for resuscitation. At the Town Hall a whole army of women supported by the municipality, was permanently kept, who were deputed to 'lay out' the corpse etc. one woman arrived at the same time as the doctor and prepared the body to be placed in a coffin and thence removed to the mortuary within 12 hours (6 hours if contagious). There, a room with entrance of glass doors, allowed observation from visitor or supervisor. Therein are three rows, twenty sarcophagi, fixed in a sloping position, the slabs on which the bodies rest are supplied with a zinc trench, filled with an antiseptic fluid. At the head of each coffin a rod is fixed, from which falls a cord having a metal ring at its extremity. Any movement of the ring on the body's finger activates a system of bells to alert the caretaker in his office.

Facilities for mortuary or postmortem examination, by comparison, were primitive in England. Of the 28 London Boroughs only 3 were declared as having 'good' mortuary accommodation. Elsewhere improvements were 'under consideration'.

This book has countless examples of reported premature burial or 'near misses' from several countries, many being observation or hearsay. It does, however, seem to have brought this subject into public debate and cases are recorded today of such occurrences.

A Waiting Mortuary, as described. Note the numbering, the sloping slabs on which the bodies were mounted and the cord and pulley system can be seen. Flower arrangements were provided as part of the service. The body is labelled with a ticket. Temperature and ventilation are controlled. There is a caretaker who makes inspections routinely and is alerted by any bell ringing. A further medical examination then takes place before interment.

This book was presented to Dr Till by a local Gloucester GP (Dr Watson) and was the first copy I had seen. I have never found a 'first edition'. New hardback editions are available on line!

3
Summary of *The Difficulties of Dr Deguerre* Dr Walter Hadwen
Published by Daniel of London 1926
In Memory of Hadwen's son Surgeon-Lieutenant John Hadwen R. N.
M. B. B. S. B. Sc. (London) L. R. C. P. M. R. C. S.
592 Pages with sketches. and photos.

THIS BOOK combines articles in the *Abolitionist* (1913–1918) with an enactment of discussions taking part by members in the imaginary Argumentative Men's Club meeting in their Pall Mall premises. The scene is set on the occasion to celebrate their 'Founders Anniversary'. Their meeting is interrupted by the noise of demonstrators parading outside their rooms who are BUAV supporters and leaflets being pushed through the window of the meeting room. This then stimulates an agreement to debate the subject of vivisection when they next meet. The mix of members include a judge, stockbroker, Bishop, Professor of political economy, a retired Colonel, a 'settlement officer' for the London East End, an editor of a scientific journal and a Harley Street physician, 'Dr Deguerre'.

The story of their meetings at the Club and also at their respective houses involves more debate and information to be shared not only amongst themselves but also their families. It gives the author the opportunity to cast doubt on many of the accepted medical practices of the day.

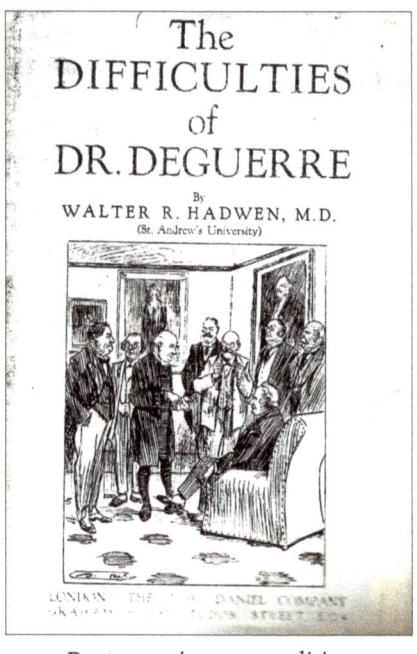

Dust cover in poor condition

Much was claimed from animal experiments but false observations and biased recording of results left the medical profession open to criticism. Personal views, self promotion and and financial gain all influenced the need for animal experimentation. There was a casual attitude in medical schools to animal experiments which were repeated in demonstrations to no advantage. Humane killing of such animals at the end of their useful purpose and similar processes in slaughter houses left the observer to worry as to how pain free such procedures really were. False information was apparent of the part played by germs in typhoid and in the origin of Malta Fever. Myxoedema research involved undue suffering amongst monkeys in the laboratory. The over diagnosis of diphtheria and use of antitoxin came into review with the revelation that the germ involved may be found on a throat swab but not necessarily that the patient had any symptoms of disease. Antitoxin was a treatment with much morbidity. Then smallpox vaccination came under scrutiny and the question of transfer of other diseases by this procedure, including syphilis, was a major concern.

Throughout the book emphasis is made of observations of the natural world and human activity that can reveal almost as much as any science laboratory and animal experiment. Often results were interpreted for the self enhancement of the experimenter's career rather than the advantage to a patient. It is cited that much animal experimentation resulted in tuberculin being produced as a treatment for tuberculosis and yet this was a failure. Inoculation experiments are debated and mention made of the large number of animals used in laboratories and that they should not be counted as just vermin. This was all a revelation to the debaters. Also many small animals had been injected with cancer material without any clear result and correlation between animal and human disease seemed unproven. Criticism of medical training and casual use of animals in laboratory demonstrations was aired. Views of abhorrence of so called 'humane' killing in slaughter houses were again expressed. The book continues to introduce controversial topics when the Club members exchange visits to each other's homes. Again, the germ theory was derided.

Dr Deguerre's wife and daughter are brought into the picture and discuss with their visitors the advantages of their living in the countryside observing Nature rather than a city full of traffic and turmoil. A city dweller, a medical researcher, had been giving Deguerre his expertise on the value of vivisection only to find that there was much more to be revealed and respected in nature's cycle of events than down a microscope. Worries are expressed that 'education' was giving the countryfolk great expectation and they feared exodus of the young to the city.

A dissertation takes place over the cause of Typhoid and claims made that many animals were used in the laboratory to discover the causal bacterium. Contentious argument took place over typhoid diagnosis inaccuracies. Statistics come under scrutiny and suspicion.

The story then includes the Colonel going on holiday to Malta and detail of Malta Fever with the inevitable argument about the use of animal experiments to discover the cause. The authorities attempts to slaughter all the goats comes under criticism. The theory of poor sanitation is put forward as the cause. The tourist's description of the capital Valetta and its history is well thought through and must reflect Hadwen's visit there. More statistics and stories are told to undermine the evidence Sir David Bruce had produced to support his theory of Goat's Milk contamination.

A new meeting of the Club was planned and discussion took place of multiple experiments on animals to establish the cause of thyroid deficiency. Evidence was put forward that thyroid deficiency as a cause of myxoedema was clinically recorded long before multiple experiments on monkeys, dogs and rabbits were performed (Prof. Kocher of Berne, Nobel Prize winner). One day the Doctor, whilst in London, was requested to return home as his daughter was ill. The family doctor had diagnosed diphtheria and concern was apparent when the question of the use of antitoxin was advised by the family doctor. However, a family member came to nurse Deguerre's daughter and made a diagnosis of quinsy which was treated successfully by fomentations rather than antitoxin. A throat swab produced the diphtheria bacillus (then known as Klebbs-Loffler). The story shows that over-diagnosis of diphtheria was common and antitoxin treatment overused with many disastrous side effects including anaphylaxis. This view was given some support by the Royal Commission investigating the subject. It was admitted that a throat swab may grow the bacillus but the patient may not ever develop the disease.

Following on from this incident Dr Deguerre and his own family doctor went on to discuss the merits of smallpox vaccination and its effectiveness. A case was described which brought to light the symptoms of a child resembled a syphilitic eruption like a chancre, but the accusation was that this was caused by calf-lymph contamination. The toxicity of Salvarsan (an arsenical compound) in treating syphilis is exposed in discussion. It would seem such a drug causes death and paralysis itself. In a further chapter colleagues discussed operative surgery and the theory of asepsis and antiseptic techniques were revealed.

Dr Deguerre then arranges to visit and see the conditions of animals in an experimental laboratory. This research unit is run by a self-opinionated bacteriologist, a Dr Simkin. He reveals that Government inspectors have little authority, control or knowledge of the laboratory animal conditions. In the research unit he meets Dr Drew, a Naval Surgeon who is gaining further training. Dr Drew is shortly introduced to Deguerre's daughter at their country home. Darwin and evolution and Christianity make for a detailed exchange of ideas. Further conversation embraces the subject of Harvey's description of circulation resulting from vivisection experiments. The question was, could not the 'discovery' come from observation and the human post mortem room?

The Deguerre family and Dr Drew attended morning service and the Preacher was Degurre's friend, the Bishop Middlepath, and by chance it was 'animals Sunday' and he preached on kindness to animals.

One chapter deals with the alleged outbreak of plague in East Anglia (1911) involving the rat and flea bite theory of germ transmission. Dr Simkin claims total knowledge of the causes provoking earnest debate on bacteriological cause verses effectiveness of improved sanitation. The Deguerre family are distraught to find that Dr. Simkin, with whom they have differed over so many theories of disease, has been invested as a knight for his work. Not only that, but Dr. Simkin arrives at Dr Deguerre's house and unexpectedly proposes to his daughter who has no hesitation in refusing.

The Argumentative Club reassembles and immediately wades into the reports of anti-rabies vaccine treatment and resultant high mortality rates thereafter. Once more the germ theory and classification of diseases are attacked. Influenza was said to be caused by a micrococcus, virus research was still an unknown quantity.

Dr Deguerre was elected President of his Teaching Hospital Medico-Shirurgical Society following on the presidential year of Dr Simkin, his knighted friend, bacteriologist and vivisector. The influence of discussions in the past years had made Deguerre certain that vivisection had little to offer in the progress of science and so he would be heading into controversy, enmity amongst his colleagues and his integrity challenged.

Dr Drew visits the Deguerre household before his next Naval posting and the question of cause and research into 'Sleeping Sickness' is explored. The next subject to be investigated at the Argumentative Club is Rabies, Hydrophobia and Tetanus. Evidence is quoted that inoculations had not saved a single life and once more Pasteur's work vilified. However, Dr Drew proposes to Deguerre's daughter and she accepts, their views on animal welfare having gelled. But the Bishop, on a visit to Deguerre's home raises the question of drug experiments on animals and their relevance and predictability for human therapy.

Malaria and mosquitos, and also the evidence behind mosquito transmission of yellow fever are mentioned before the book finishes with the last meeting of the Argumentative Club with unanimous support for the anti-vivisection cause.

4
Summary of *First Impressions of America* Dr Hadwen
1921 Hutchinson and Co. Illustrated
320 pages forming the basis for articles published in the Gloucester *Citizen*

THIS TRAVELOGUE was, in part, published in the local newspaper, the Gloucester *Citizen*, with the idea of the reader being able to envisage the major cities and places of interest visited by the author but the reader was unlikely to have the opportunity to see for themselves. The excitement generated on seeing New York starts the adventure and concise descriptions including plenty of relevant statistic of buildings make an interesting comparison for anyone travelling to the USA as a tourist today.

The book does not give tribute to any illustrator and the 'mini sketches' are a delightful addition to the prose. For the first time Hadwen mentions having a Kodak camera and I am reasonably certain that, once home, Hadwen used photographs to copy and create the illustrations.

At the age of 67 years Hadwen sailed on the *Mauretania* of the Cunard Line to New York on 30th April 1921, sailing from Southampton to New York via Cherbourg. According to the Cunard passenger list he travelled 2nd Class in Cabin 104 (of 345 available). Before he travelled Hadwen realised that regulations about vaccination might exclude him from entering USA, confirmed at an interview with the American Consul. Thomas Cook agent sought advice and Hadwen decided to take a chance. At Cherbourg he discovered that the regulation relating to vaccination applied only to foreign ports, and that passengers from England were excluded.

The places he visited were planned around an invitation to lecture on the subject of antivivisection, animal welfare and no doubt anti vaccination. Almost certainly this tour was sponsored by admirers to defray expenses and offer hospitality. He lectured in Washington, Boston, Philadelphia, Chicago and New York and many more. He was interviewed by reporters in New York where he gave a presentation in the iconic Plaza Hotel supported by the local Antivivisection Society.

The tour apparently was of some ten weeks duration and we do not know the actual planned route Hadwen embarked upon once in USA but many thousand miles were covered. The starting point was his first view of Manhattan Island, the thrill of the skyscrapers and the Statue of Liberty. What seem like irrelevant observations make for lighter reading, noting the 170 page Sunday newspaper with colour and that daily papers were 'thrown' on the frontage of houses not 'posted'. House plots were open plan without walls, gates or railings or hedges. Roads seemed to be remarkably straight and fuel only cost one shilling per gallon. He described Central Park as being a perfect country scene. In contrast he admired the Railway Station architecture.

He was disappointed to learn that William Rockefeller used some of his fortune to found an institute that was a centre for experiments on living animals.

He comments on class distinction by wealth and colour prejudice. He added that white families were gradually cutting down on their black servants or housemaids, this in turn creating unemployment and tensions. In his text he uses the words 'Negro' and 'Darkie'. The invention of the Hoover vacuum reduced the need for staff and many wealthy families just had a gardener. He observed that the progress intellectually of the negro would eventually have consequences for society. He attended a variety of church services, including the Cathedral of St. John the Divine and St. Patrick's Cathedral. In contrast he attended a Christian Science church where he noted there were no poor people. He enjoyed the joyous hymn singing in an evangelical mission hall.

He describes Boston as 'The home of Literacy', Philadelphia as 'The Quaker city'. Hadwen visited Washington twice and he was able to explore the Capitol and National monument also the debating chambers of House of Representatives and the Senate. He was invited to speak to the Senate appointed committee gathering evidence for a forthcoming debate and Bill for the Abolition of the Vivisection of Dogs. This meeting was interrupted before completion after four hours due to the German Peace Bill coming before the Senate and requiring all Senate members to attend and vote. However he did have a very acceptable vegetarian meal in one of the dining halls.

He went on, by invitation to the White House and visited the President's Room, the date is not recorded. He had an interview with President Harding putting forward his view of total abolition of vivisection and had a discussion with Mrs Harding who appeared to support prosecuting anyone responsible for animal cruelty.

Between the major cities, transport was mainly by train and he describes the sleeping car which he occupied for nearly a week. He enjoyed the facility of the observation car but the open air platform was spoilt by the constant blowing of tobacco smoke in his face and the pervading smell of peppermint from chewing gum.

His tour included going by train to Buffalo and then on to Niagara Falls and viewing the amazing vista from Prospect Point and mentioning the whirlpool rapids where Capt. Webb died attempting to swim across.

His route is difficult to ascertain but he takes in a journey through Iowa, Illinois Utah, Kansas, Colorado and New Mexico and this long train journey was a fruitful experience as there was a young Mormon lady who spoke openly about her beliefs. He was impressed by their abstention from smoking and alcohol. He was guided round the temple grounds and the tabernacle seating 10,000 people. He describes the local industry and fruit and dairy farms. Eventually he arrives in California where he was a speaker at many meetings. At some point he is able to divert to the Grand Canyon via Williams where there he takes the historic train journey to the Canyon. He takes a mule trek down the Bright Angel trail, which he finds a difficult and frightening experience. He states that there were five men and one girl on mules with a cowboy guide, the trail is seven miles long via the Devil's Corkscrew 6000 ft descent.

His next destination was to travel in a friend's car to the West Coast, via the majestic Sierra Nevada, to an area of Los Angeles called Venice on the Pacific Coast. He describes the similarities to Italy's Venice, the

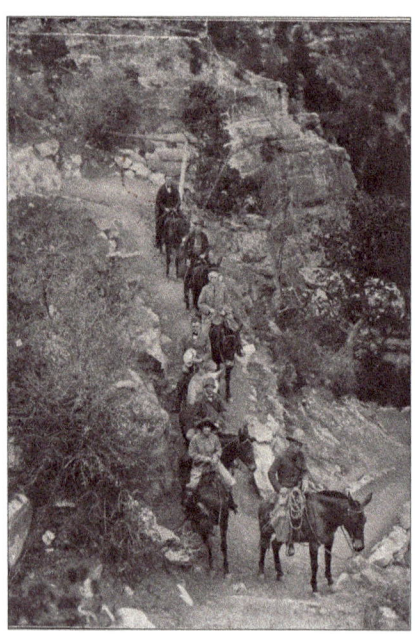

Original in archive

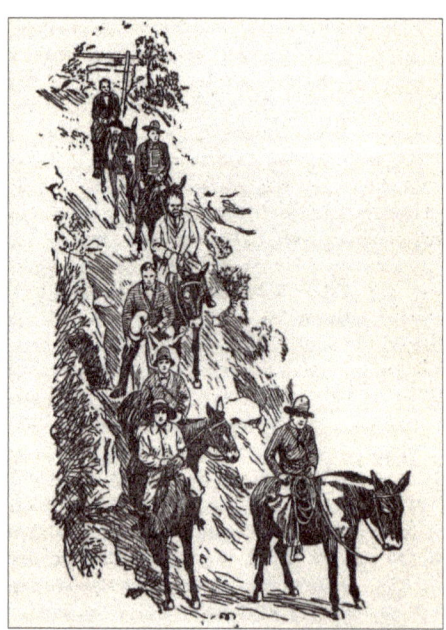

Sketch by Hadwen in his Book

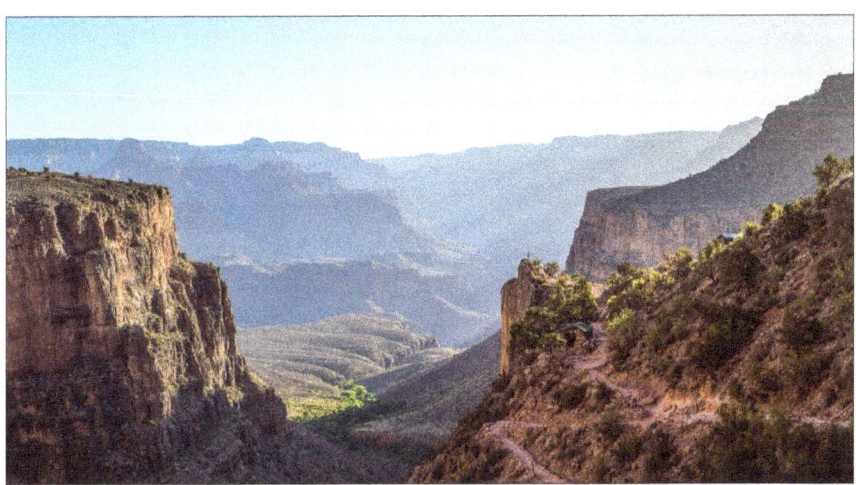
Bright Angel Trail as it is today

bridges across the canals and the gondolas but no Doge's Palace and the copy St Mark's Plaza disappointed. This was amply compensated for by his observation of the ladies on the beach 'tis true they each had on a skin tight coloured jersey, which reaches from just above the breasts to the hip joint' and further comment ensued about the appropriate dress of the fairer sex and beachwear!. Amazingly he actually seemed to rest, stopping for a picnic on the beach. His friend's daughter had accompanied them. She showed him some dull looking stones she had collected on the beach, they are described as 'Californian Jewels'. As he left his friend in California the little girl presented a little tin box and she said 'put them in your pocket, it is a memento of a pleasant day's outing'. The stones were described as 'light coloured ones are moonstones, the red ones are sardonyx and the greenish colour one is jasper' most were polished. This keepsake has survived and handed down the family and stones are illustrated, but maybe not the complete original set.

Los Angeles had an active Antivivisection Society and it was they who originally invited and supported Hadwen's tour and covered all travel expenses.

Next, he arrives in San Diego, the 'Harbour of the Sun', an example of the string of Spanish Mission Stations along the Pacific

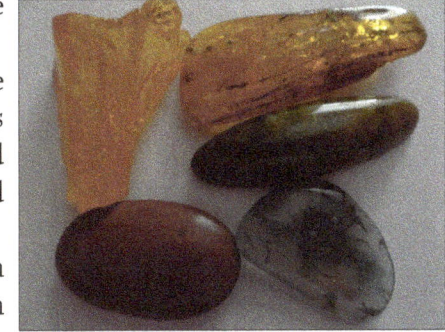
The stones from the beach at Venice as a present to Hadwen

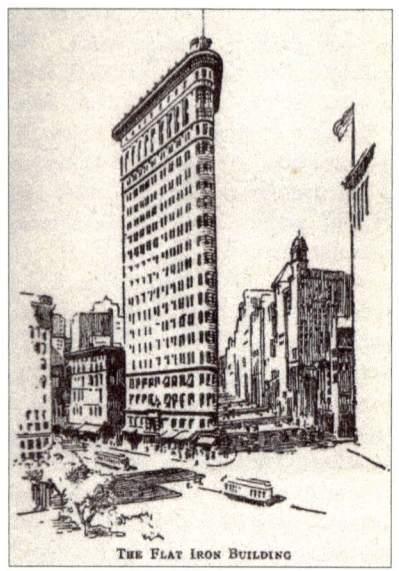
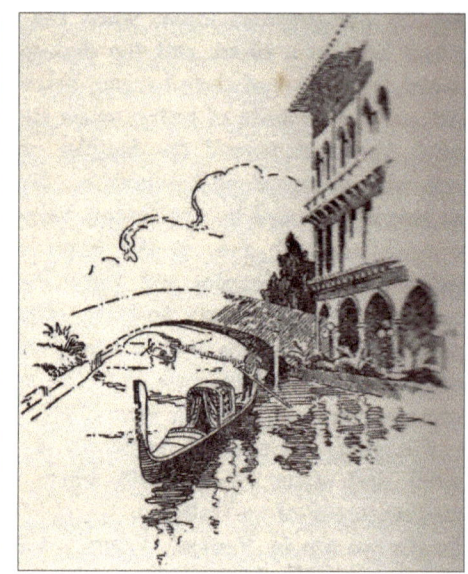

'Flatiron Building' New York City   Venice, Los Angeles
Sketches in his book

Coast. It was founded 1769. He marvelled at the orange groves with their golden fruit and the numerous palm trees. Walnut and Olive trees abounded and the colours of fields of beet and bright green alfa-alfa completed a contrast. Land was originally bought up for one shilling an acre by an entrepreneur. He was captivated by the city and its history.

His last city visited in the book was San Francisco and the 'Golden Gate' which describes the strait between the headlands of the Francisco and Marin peninsulas. He was not to know that the famous bridge would be constructed to connect the two in 1937. He admired all he saw and was passionate about the whole area and the sublime sunsets.

However there is no mention of his visit to his son's grave in San Diego which one can only assume he wanted kept as a private memory..

There is no 'final chapter' or 'conclusion' to the book but the last paragraph gives you an impression of Hadwen's feelings as quoted on interview by a newspaper reporter. 'America is a great and fascinating country, full of marvellous revelations and possibilities: it is possessed by a wonderful, kind-hearted, resourceful and intensely clever people, and I am as proud of it and fond of it as you are'.

According to passenger listing, Hadwen returned from New York to Southampton on 12 July, 1921 on the Cunard liner *Aquitania*.

BIBLIOGRAPHY, BOOKS AND REFERENCES

Books

Arnold, Catherine, 2018, *Pandemic 1918*, Michael O'Mara Books.
Beggs, Martin, 2006, *One Hundred Years in Southgate Street*, Qwertyop,Slad.
Bondeson, Jan, 2001, *Buried Alive*. Norton & Co.
British Medical Association, 1909, *Secret Remedies*, BMA.
British Medical Association, 1912, *More Secret Remedies*, BMA.
Burch, Druin, 2007, *Digging up the Dead*, Chatto & Windus.
Durbach,Nadia, 2005, *Bodily Matters*, Duke University Press.
Glynn, Ian and Jennifer, 2004, *The Life and Death of Smallpox*, Profile Books.
Hadwen, Walter R, 1921, *First Impressions of America*, Hutchinson.
Hadwen, Walter R, 1926, *The Difficulties of Dr.Deguerre*, C.W.Daniel Co.
Hopley, Emma, 1998, *Campaigning Against Cruelty*, Regent Publishing Services.
Kidd, B.E., and Richards, M.E., 1933, *Hadwen of Gloucester*, John Murray.
Offit, Paul, 2011, *Deadly Choices*. Basic Books/ Perseus Group.
Roach, Mary, 2003, *Stiff, The Curious Lives of Human Cadavers*, Viking.
Tebb, William, and Vollum, Edward P., 1905, *Premature Burial, and how it may be prevented*; 2nd edition by Walter Hadwen, Swan Sonnenschein.
Williams, Gareth, 2010, *Angel of Death, The Story of Smallpox*, Palgrave Macmillan.

Reports

BUAV, 1924, *Verbatim Report of the Trail and Acquittal of Dr W R Hadwen.JP*, 65 pages.
BUAV, 1924, 'The Trial for Manslaughter,Dr W R Hadwen', *The Abolitionist*, no.12, vol. XXV.

Anti-Immunisation, Anti-Vaccination and Smallpox.

Hadwen, Walter R., 1896, *The Case Against Vaccination: an address*, Gloucester BUAV, 37 pages.
Hadwen, Walter R., 1896, *The Outbreak of Smallpox in Gloucester and its causes*, reprint from *Bristol Mercury*, National Anti-vaccination League.

Hadwen, Walter R., 1898, *Smallpox at Gloucester: a Reply to Dr Coupland's Report*, Anti-Vaccination League, 3 pages.
Hadwen, Walter R., 1902, *The Vaccination Delusion* (lecture), Liverpool Anti-Vaccination League, 31 pages.
Hadwen, Walter R., 1903 *The Vivisection Question*, BUAV, 31 pages.
Hadwen, Walter R., 1903, *Lecture*, The Imperial Vaccination League, London, 28 pages.
Hadwen, Walter R., 1912, *Tuberculin as a treatment for Consumption*, BUAV, 7 pages.
Hadwen, Walter R., 1925, *Antitoxin Treatment of Diphtheria*, BUAV, 25 pages.
Hadwen, Walter R., 1931, *Diphtheria Immunization*, BUAV.
Hadwen, Walter R., *'New Tuberculin': The Latest Medical Quackery*, BUAV. 9 pages.
Millard,C. Killick, 1950, *Smallpox and Vaccination, My Confession of Faith*, National Anti-Vaccination League, 17 pages.
National Anti-Vaccination League, 1924, *Vaccination at Work: What it is and What it does*, 4th edition. (Misc. authors), 40 pages.
National Anti-Vaccination League (undated), *Vaccine Virus, What is it?*, 1 page.
National Anti-Vaccination League (undated), *Tyranny of Vaccination*, 3 pages.
National Anti-vaccination League (undated), *Diphtheria Immunisation: Useless, Injurious and Unnecessary*, 2 pages.
Pickering, J.N.O., 1896, *The Small-Pox Epidemic in Gloucester and Water Cure*, (privately published), 52 pages.
Rose,Charles,1983, *How to Cure and Prevent Small-Pox*, 11 pages.

Anti-Vivisection.

Hadwen, Walter R., (undated), *The Cult Of the Vivisector*, BUAV, 7 pages.
Hadwen, Walter R., 1902, *Vivisection Practices in English Laboratories*, BUAV, 16 pages.
Hadwen, Walter R., 1903, *The Medical View of the Vivisection Question: address at Assembly Rooms, Bath*, BUAV.
Hadwen Walter R., 1906, *The Humour of the Vivisector*, BUAV, 8 pages.
Hadwen, Walter R., 1907, *Should Vivisection be Abolished?: Glossop Debate between Dr Thomas Eastham and Dr W Hadwen*, BUAV, 24 pages.
Hadwen, Walter R., 1908, *Is Vivisection Immoral, Cruel, Useless, Unscientific?: Report on Debate, Shrewsbury, Stephen Paget FRCS v DR.W. Hadwen*, BUAV, 27 pages.
Hadwen, Walter R., 1912, *Review of Report of Royal Commission on Vivisection*, BUAV, 23 pages.
Hadwen, Walter R., 1914, *Jennerism and Pasteurism*, BUAV, 15 pages.
Hadwen, Walter R., 1917, *Vivisection under the Insurance Act*, BUAV, 21 pages.
Hadwen, Walter R., 1917, *Vivisection in Liverpool*, BUAV, 6 pages.
Hadwen, Walter R., 1917, *Recent British Vivisections*, BUAV, 29 pages.
Hadwen, Walter R., 1926, *The VivIsection Problem Today*, BUAV, 7 pages.
Hadwen, Walter R., (undated), *The Bishop of Birmingham's Views on Modern*

Medicine and the Miracles of Christ, BUAV, 15 pages.
Hadwen, Walter R., (undated), *The Blunders of a Bishop*, BUAV, 8 pages.
Hadwen, Walter R., *Urging the Rejection of the Dog's Protection Bill: Note to 9 Members of Parliament*, BUAV, 4 pages.
Hadwen, Walter R., *The Dogs 'Fourteen Points: Reply to Critics of Dogs Bill*, BUAV, 7 pages.
Hadwen, Walter R., 1914, *The Dogs Bill: Report on Debate, Dr Chapple MP MD v Dr W. Hadwen, Held in the House of Commons*, BUAV, 38 pages.
Hadwen, Walter R., (undated), *The International Medical Congress, What has been gained by it?*, BUAV, 19 pages.
Hadwen, Walter R., and Paget, Stephen, 1910, *A Vivisection Controversy: Report of Discussion and Correspondence*, BUAV, 44 pages.
Hadwen, Walter R., (undated), *Tuberculosis and Cow's Milk*, BUAV, 18 pages.
Hadwen, Walter R,, (undated), *Rats and Fleas: The Riddle of the Plague*, BUAV, 14 pages.
Hadwen, Walter R., (undated), *Antisepsis or Asepsis: an Explanation*, BUAV, 8 pages.
Hadwen, Walter R., (undated), *Pasteur and Pasteurism*. BUAV, 32 pages.
Hadwen, Walter R., 1914, *Experiments on Living Animals: Address at Newcastle*, BUAV, 28 pages.
Hadwen, Walter R., 1917, *Vivisection in Liverpool*, BUAV.
Hadwen, Walter R.,1923, *The relationship between Insanitation and Disease: Paper read before the Institute of Sanitary Engineers*, BUAV, 16 pages.
Hadwen, Walter R., 1930, *Tortured Motherhood*, BUAV, 2 pages.
Hadwen, Walter R. 1930, *The Modern Medicine Man: How he manufactures his Vaccines and serums*, BUAV, 11 pages.
Hadwen, Walter R., *The Real Truth about Vivisection: Reply to attack on the New York anti-vivisection Society in 1921*, BUAV 36pages (first published in New York, and reprinted).

Miscellaneous.

Hadwen, Walter R., 1912, *Reply to Prof.Schafer on 'The Origin of Life'*. BUAV, 12 pages.
Hadwen, Walter R., 1916, *The Institution of the Lord's Supper*, (privately published), 58 pages.
Hadwen, Walter R., 1931, *A Sermon on Vivisection: St Cuthbert's Church, York*, BUAV

ACKNOWLEDGEMENTS

Marvin Begg and his book *One Hundred Years in Southgate Street* with detail of Dr Hadwen's part in the origin of Albion Hall and his participation as a teacher and preacher.

Cruelty Free International (formerly BUAV) Dr Katy Tyler, Director.

Animal Free Research UK (Formerly Dr. Hadwen Trust).

Special Collections, Bristol University for details of Hadwen's prizes.

Dr Toby Thacker, Senior Lecturer in Modern European History, Cardiff for information on 1923 epidemic in Gloucester and for advice and assistance.

Paul Drinkwater for access to information he collected for lecture on Dr. Hadwen at the Gloucester History Festival 2018.

Dr John Chandler, Historian and Publisher.

Heather Forbes, Head of Archives Service, Gloucestershire Archives.

Dr Martin O'Dell for proof reading, advice and interest in local medical history.

Nick Darien-Jones for allowing me access to Hadwen's house 'Hillside'.

Dr Susan L Speaker, PhD, Historian, National Library of Medicine, Bethesda, Maryland, USA

INDEX

This is a selective index of the principal places, people and organisations. Places visited by Hadwen on his tours and described in chapter 12 and appendix 4 have not been indexed

Abolitionist - publication 57-59, 130, 135,
Albion Hall, Gloucester 34
Anti-Vaccination League 18, 61, 69
Apothecaries, Licentiate, Society of 11
Axbridge Petty Sessions
    Refusing vaccination case 13
    Dog Poisoning case 19

Barton Street Surgery, Gloucester 31
Best, Gertrude, Choir Leader 35
Bibby, Dr. MOH Gloucester City 94, 95, 100
Blackwood, Sir Arthur 10
BMA 33, 45, 62, 71, 122,
BMJ 33, 59, 71, 82, 104, 142, 143
Booth, General William 67
Bond, Dr Francis 44, 51
Bristol Mercury Letter 46-53
Bristol University Medical School and Prizes 21
British Medical Association (BMA) 33, 45, 62, 71, 122,
British Medical Journal (BMJ) 33, 59, 71, 82, 104, 142, 143
British Union against Vivisection 57
Bruce, David. Maj.Gen. RAMC 71
Brucellosis (Malta Fever) 71
Brunswick House, Gloucester 29
BUAV 57
Burnham-on-Sea 21

Campbell, Dr John, MOH 55
Campbell, Dr John D.C., partner 148
Chadwick, Edwin 50
Chillingham Castle 125
Citizen newspaper 54, 78, 81, 132, 147
Cobbe, Frances Power 57, 59
Coupland's Report 55

Crimson Cross Remedy 143
Cripps, Sir Stafford 148

Davidson, Dr William, MOH 95
Difficulties of Dr Deguerre, book 85, 177-81
Dr Coupland's Report 55
Dr Hadwen Trust for Humane Research 154
Duckworth Pharmacy 31, 140

East End Tabernacle, Gloucester 31
Ellis, Dr E.S., G.P. 106, 119, 158
Eulalie (Rodenhurst) 35

'Fan' Hadwen's Collie dog 11, 75
First Impressions of America, book 130, 182-6
Flu (Spanish) Pandemic 91

Glevum Way Surgery, Abbeydale, Gloucester 149
Gloucester Aircraft Co. Brockworth 95, 102, 152/3
Gloucester Cathedral, Jenner statue 29
Gloucester Medical and Hydropathic Association 30
Gloucester Rotary Club 132
Gothic Cottages/ Cholera Hospital 28
Graham, Dr E. 110

Hadwen, Gracie 19, 30, 35, 61, 85, 138
Hadwen, John (brother) 73
Hadwen, John (Jack) (son) 13, 83
Hadwen, Walter,
    City Councillor 56
    Funeral 135
    Licentiate, Society of Apothecaries 11
    Magistrate 56

Marriage 12
Memorial 137
President BUAV 60
Sanitary Committee 56
School Board 36
Voice recording 72, 78
Will 138
Harding, Warren, President USA 131
Harral, Dr and Mrs, and Alice 12
Headlam, Dr Arthur, Bishop of Gloucester 100
Highbridge, Somerset 12
'Hillside', Pitchcombe 37-42
Horsley, Dr James 147
Humane Research, Dr Hadwen Trust for 154
Hydropathic centre 30

Isle of Man Legislative Council 71

Kidd, Beatrice 59, 86, 120, 129, 135

Jenner/Jennerism 27
Jenner Museum 156
Jenner statue, Gloucester Cathedral 29

Lancaster Royal Grammar School 9, 155
Lancaster, HMS 85-88
Lannett, isolation Hospital 26
Licentiate Society of Apothecaries 11
Lustgarten, Edgar 104

Malta Fever (Brucellosis) 71
Man, Isle of, Legislative Council 71
Medical Research Council 63
MD Qualification 23
Morris, Dr Donald 148

National anti-vaccination League 53
Nelson Street Mission Hall, Gloucester 35

Order of the Cross 148
Over Isolation Hospital 28, 94

Park Road Surgery, Gloucester 31, 129,

Pharmacy, Highbridge 12, 20
Plymouth Brethren 11, 20
Poor Law Guardians, Gloucester 27, 44
Premature Burial, book 56, 78, 171-7
Public Health Act 71

Queen Victoria 62

Recordings, voice, by Hadwen 72, 78
Rodenhurst, Eulalie 35
Rodenhurst, Una (née Hadwen) 13, 126, 134, 149
Royal Berkshire Hospital, Reading 10
Royal Commission on Vaccination 28
Royal Commission on Vivisection 62, 69
Royal Marine Infirmary, Woolwich 9

St. Agnew Hospital, San Diego 87
St. Michael's Surgery, Gloucester 150
Sanitary Committee, Gloucester 56
Secret Remedies, BMA 141
Shaw, George Bernard 61-62, 67
Smallpox
  in Gloucester 1896 36
  'Smallpox' scare 1923 92
  outbreak Bradford 1962 155
  outbreak Birmingham, 1978 156
Spanish Flu Pandemic 91

Tankerville, Countess Leonora 123, 137
Tankerville, Earl of 69, 123,
Tebb, William 18, 56

Vaccinations Act 1853 36
Vaccination Enquirer 18
van Zyl, Dr Margery 148
Variola Minor/ Alastrim 92
Victoria, Queen 62
Voice recordings by Hadwen 72

Wakefield, Sir Humphry Bt. 156
Wesley, John 68, 141
Widden Street School, Gloucester 36
Wild Cattle, Chillingham 126, 156
Woolwich 10

www.ingramcontent.com/pod-product-compliance
Lightning Source LLC
Chambersburg PA
CBHW040301170426
43193CB00021B/2974